Heal Yourself With Sunlight

Andreas Moritz

Other books and products by Andreas Moritz:

The Amazing Liver and Gallbladder Flush

Timeless Secrets of Health and Rejuvenation

Cancer Is Not a Disease

Lifting the Veil of Duality

It's Time to Come Alive

Simple Steps to Total Health

Heart Disease No More!

Diabetes—No More!

Ending the AIDS Myth

Feel Great, Lose Weight

Vaccine-Nation (July 2010)

Hear the Whispers, Live Your Dream

Sacred Santémony

Ener-Chi Art & Ener-Chi Ionized Stones

All of the above are available at www.ener-chi.com,
www.amazon.com, and other online or physical bookstores.

Heal Yourself With Sunlight

Andreas Moritz

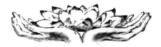

Your Health is in Your Hands

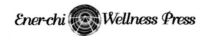

Ener-chi Wellness Press

For Reasons of Legality

The author of this book, Andreas Moritz, does not advocate the use of any particular form of health care but believes that the facts, figures, and knowledge presented herein should be available to every person concerned with improving his or her state of health. Although the author has attempted to give a profound understanding of the topics discussed and to ensure accuracy and completeness of any information that originates from any other source than his own, he and the publisher assume no responsibility for errors, inaccuracies, omissions, or any inconsistency herein. Any slights of people or organizations are unintentional. This book is not intended to replace the advice and treatment of a physician who specializes in the treatment of diseases. Any use of the information set forth herein is entirely at the reader's discretion. The author and publisher are not responsible for any adverse effects or consequences resulting from the use of any of the preparations or procedures described in this book. The statements made herein are for educational and theoretical purposes only and are mainly based upon Andreas Moritz's own opinion and theories. You should always consult with a health care practitioner before taking any dietary, nutritional, herbal or homeopathic supplement, or beginning or stopping any therapy. The author is not intending to provide any medical advice, or offer a substitute thereof, and make no warranty, expressed or implied, with respect to any product, device or therapy, whatsoever. Except as otherwise noted, no statement in this book has been reviewed or approved by the United States Food & Drug Administration or the Federal Trade Commission. Readers should use their own judgment or consult a holistic medical expert or their personal physicians for specific applications to their individual problems.

ISBN: 978-0-9792757-3-9
1st Edition (pocket book): April 2007
2nd Edition (expanded, revised, regular size): April 2010
Published by Ener-Chi Wellness Press – Ener-chi.com, United States of America

Cover Design/Artwork (Ener-Chi Art, Oil on Canvas): By Andreas Moritz

Table of Contents

Introduction – Sunlight Medicine of Nature   vii

1. The Sun – The Ultimate Source of Life on Earth   1

2. The Miraculous Healing Powers of Ultraviolet Light   5

3. Can UV-Radiation Prevent and Cure Skin Cancer?   11

4. The More UV, the Less Cancer   23

5. Now Even Doctors and Scientists Say: "It's Not True!"   31

6. Skin Cancer Caused By Sun Protection   35

7. Deficient Sunlight – A Death Trap   59

8. Pittas –Watch Out!   68

9. No Sun, No Health!   73

10. Sunlight Prevents Cancer, Multiple Sclerosis,
Heart Disease, Arthritis, Diabetes   84

11. The Sun Cuts Cancer Risk by Half or More!   99

12. The Amazing Sunlight/Exercise Combination   107

13. What Makes the Sun so "Dangerous"
- The Fat Connection!   120

14. What Really Burns and Damages the Skin   145

15. Guidelines for Increasing Sun Exposure   164

16. The Ancient Practice of Sun Gazing   168

About the author Andreas Moritz   172

Other books, products and services by Andreas Moritz   174

Index   185

INTRODUCTION
Sunlight – Medicine of Nature

The first, most likely thing to pop up in your mind, when you hear the word 'medicine' is a pill in a plastic box from a pharmacy and a doctor's prescription.

But in truth, not all medicines come in pills with prescriptions.

There are more fundamental, more basic, more essential healing substances and energies. These are freely available to every one of us in the vast pharmacy called nature, where you are your own doctor and your own body sends out little prescriptions to you every now and then when things aren't in order. These prescriptions are signs and symptoms that are subjectively appreciable.

Let me give you a small analogy. When you are dehydrated, your body tells you that it needs water. Thirst is what you subjectively experience. Your mouth feels dry and you yourself know that a drink of water (a free and natural substance) will fix the problem. You don't need a medical professional to tell you that. You just instinctively know that water alone, will do the job.

Likewise, medicines are not limited to the conventional pills or tablets or capsules with names, dosages, expiry dates and barcodes.

There are many other indispensable, reliable and abundant natural remedies - the most vital of them all, being sunlight. It is one among those countless potent remedies in nature's apothecary.

Sadly, the sun has been maligned as the cause for, rather than the solution to many of our problems. Let me illustrate this fact: you are flipping through pages of a magazine, one among the many stacked up in the corner of the waiting room. A young woman with a somber expression meaningfully holds up a framed photograph of a pretty smiling blonde. "My sister accidently killed herself. She died of skin cancer", goes the headline of the public service announcement.

Shock and sympathy sweep in. Fear and anxiety creep in. The message is alarming. 'Make sun safety a way of life', is the appeal and you panic. You certainly don't want to be a victim of solar assault, a sad photo in a frame. So your first reaction is to hop into a shop without delay and purchase sunscreen, the legitimate protection from the dangers of sunlight, as you have been made to believe.

But wait a minute!

All things must not be taken at face value. You have just been deceived by a cleverly crafted lie.

The sun is NOT your foe, it is your friend. You exist because it exists. You are simply ASKING for trouble by abandoning the natural and favoring the unnatural. You are sacrificing your health and possibly even your life for the economic gains of people you do not even know.

Disturbing as it appears, the misleading 'public service announcement' in the magazine was actually put forward by a prominent charitable cancer organization and was sponsored by a company with a direct financial interest. In other words, it is nothing but an advertisement that was financed by one of the leading sunscreen manufacturing companies. It featured in several women's magazines all through the summer. Allow me to quote the precise warning in the advertisement: "if left unchecked, skin cancer can be fatal". It also urges people to "use sunscreen, cover up and watch for skin changes".

Let's come to the shameful truth. With a little investigation, you will learn that the woman in the picture is a professional model, not a skin cancer victim. Also, the poignant message implied that those who die of skin cancer die because of their own injudiciousness, happens to lack any clear supporting evidence.

To many, this advertisement is an unjustifiable attempt at manipulation of public opinion. To many others it is an absolute breach of trust and faith that has been innocently placed in an organization that is believed to have the public's best interests at heart. The incident raised a fair deal of concern among academicians and common people alike especially since the same organization became the nation's wealthiest charity largely through its public relations acumen. The fact that the principal creator of the organization is still remembered for his devastatingly effective cigarette advertising campaigns incorporating the slogan "Reach for a Lucky [cigarette] instead of a sweet" does nothing to restore people's faith in the establishment.

Yes, the organization is partially correct in telling the public that skin cancer is fatal because there indeed are lethal kinds of skin cancers called malignant melanomas. But these deadly forms of skin cancer comprise only 6 percent of the overall number of skin cancer cases in the U.S. each year; the remaining 94 percent are NOT life-threatening. Unfortunately most people have a very vague comprehension of the difference between the rare but potentially fatal forms of skin cancer and the benign ones. It appears that several organizations aim at exploiting this lack of awareness on the part of the common man.

The more common types of skin cancer - basal cell and squamous cell skin tumors - are not even considered as cancer in the National Cancer Institute's SEER database, which gathers epidemiological information on the incidence and survival rates of cancer in the U.S. Basal cell and squamous cell skin cancers rarely metastasize, are almost always readily cured, and very rarely ever kill anyone. No one has ever heard or spoken of these more common cancers as "deadly squamous cell carcinoma" or "lethal basal cell carcinoma".

To randomly warn the general public, that sun exposure causes deadly skin cancers which mercilessly claim lives, without distinguishing between rare fatal melanomas and the much more common, curable skin tumors, seems like a deliberate effort made to instill fear if not to terrorize people.

The motive is quite visibly to promote sales of sunscreens and other sun protection. It is a monetary motive.

The truth: sunscreen, at best, can only prevent sunburn. It cannot and does not prevent the RAREST and only true fatal form of skin cancer - malignant melanoma. No conclusive association has ever been made between sunburns and melanoma. How then is it logical to suggest that sunscreens can save you from death by skin cancer? In fact, studies suggest that people are at greater risk of developing melanomas by the use of sunscreens.

In this book I wish to make people look beyond the contrivances and lies about sun exposure that have been thrown in our faces, and more importantly, to help people realize the countless benefits of sunlight. You deserve to know the truth. In today's world awareness is everything.

Andreas Moritz, April 2010

'Dare to reach out your hand into the darkness, to pull another into the light.'

CHAPTER 1:
The Sun - The Ultimate Source of Life on Earth

Sunlight is the most crucial biological requirement for survival and perpetuation. We owe our very existence to it. If there was no sun, there would be no earth and so no life, no mankind.

The very first life forms on planet earth employed sunlight as the raw material for survival. These were photosynthetic organisms, autotrophic organisms. Even today, after ages of evolution, they persist. We have all evolved from these primitive sun-dependent life forms. Although we have emerged as the most complex beings, we have still retained a very basic dependence on sunlight. We perish without it.

Regular exposure of our body to the germicidal wavelength of ultraviolet light (UV) of the sun successfully controls germs, mites, molds, bacteria, and viruses.

UV radiation is so potent that it is even used in industries as a method for sterilization of water, foods, instruments, etc. Many bacteria, viruses and viable substances are killed with prolonged exposure under direct sunlight. A specific example is Neisseria gonorrhea which dies in the open air under hours of exposure to sunlight; the same is true for lots of other pathogenic bacteria.

Did you know, for example, that sunlight kills bacteria and is quite capable of doing so even when it has passed through window glass? Also, are you aware that sunlit hospital wards have lesser bacteria in them than dark wards?

Its powerful, immune stimulating effect makes sunlight one of the most important disease-inhibitors. But this is only one of the many benefits sunlight has to offer for enhancing and sustaining human health.

The sun is the only true source of energy on planet Earth. It provides the perfect amount of energy for plants to synthesize all of the products required for growth and reproduction.

1

Energy can only be converted from one form to another. Solar energy is stored in plants. We consume these plants and the potential energy stored within them. The same energy is then converted into other forms of energy within our bodies.

The sun's energy is stored by plants in the form of carbohydrates, proteins and fat. When ingested, plant foods provide us with the vital energy we need in order to lead active and healthy lives. The processes of digestion, assimilation, and metabolism of food in the body are mainly used to break down, transfer, store, and utilize these various forms of encapsulated solar energy.

The lowest level of the food chain, where foods are manufactured directly by sunlight, makes available to us the most sun energy. In other words, plants, which are at the base of the food pyramid, are the richest in solar energy. In contrast, products that are high up in the food chain contain little or no sun energy and are practically useless, if not harmful, for the body. These include products made from dead animals, fish, junk foods and microwave foods, frozen, irradiated, genetically engineered[1], and other highly processed foods.

Wood, fuel, and minerals, too, are merely various forms of locked-up sun energy. They are solar energy power houses. Solar energy is limitless unlike non-renewable sources.

The amount of energy the sun sends towards our planet is 35,000 times more than what we currently produce and consume. Indeed some part of this energy is reflected back

---

[1] In 1998 scientists have found the first evidence that genetically- modified food may damage human health. Researchers at the prestigious Rowett Research Institute in Aberdeen, U.K., found that genetically-modified foods could damage the immune systems of rats. Around 60 percent of the processed food products found in supermarkets—from hamburgers to ice cream—may contain ingredients that have been genetically tampered with.

into space but a lot of it is absorbed by the atmosphere and other elements. This energy can be easily harnessed for practical purposes. Our own bodies utilize solar energy.

All matter is 'frozen' light. Our body cells are bundles of sun energy.

The glucose and oxygen we feed them are products of the sun. We couldn't think or process a single thought without the molecules of sun-energized glucose and oxygen.

Air, which is warmed by the sun, is capable of absorbing water from the oceans while passing over them. As this moisture-laden air moves over land masses up to higher elevations, it starts to cool down and thereby releases some of its absorbed water. This water falls on the earth as rain or snow, feeding the rivers, and through them, the land and the vegetation.

Depending on its position in relation to the earth's rotation, the position of the moon, and the sun's internal cyclic activities (sun spot cycles), the sun masterminds the entire earth's climate and seasonal changes down to the smallest details, including temperature, amount of rainfall, cloud formation, periods of dryness, etc.

The planet is not a home only for human beings. The sun also has to support the growth of all the other species, including plants, animals, insects, and especially microbes, without which life here would not be possible. The mathematical complexity that stands behind a system of organization as infinitely diverse and intricate as planetary life cannot be fathomed, even by a trillion supercomputers. But the sun, without making mistakes, 'calculates' what each species - whether it is an ant, a tree, or a human being - requires in order to fulfill its evolutionary purpose and cycle.

It is no surprise then that the sun was deified by our ancestors. People all over the world, different civilizations and cultures independently worshiped the sun.

Apollo - the Roman sun deity was believed to be the God of light and healing. In ancient Greek literature, Helios has been described as the sun-god bearing an aureole, driving a chariot across the sky each day. To the ancient Egyptians, Ra was the sun - a manifestation of divinity. They believed man was born from the tears of Ra. The Chinese believed that there were 10 suns that appeared in turns. The Hindu people believed in saluting the sun by assuming certain yogic postures and chanting sacred mantras. The exercise was known as Surya Namaskar and is still performed by many today.

The electromagnetic waves generated by the sun come in a variety of lengths, which determine their specific course of action and responsibility. They range from a 0.00001 nanometer for cosmic rays (a nanometer is one billionth of a meter) to about 4,990 kilometers for electric waves. There are cosmic rays, gamma rays, x-rays, various kinds of Ultraviolet rays, the visible light spectrum consisting of seven color rays, short-wave infrared, infrared, radio waves, and electric waves. Most of these energy waves are absorbed and used for various processes in the layers of atmosphere that surround the earth.

Only a small portion of them - the electromagnetic spectrum - reach the surface of the earth. The human eye, though, can perceive just about one percent of this spectrum. Although we are unable to see any of the ultraviolet and infrared waves, they exert a very strong influence on us.

In fact, ultraviolet light has proved to be the most biologically active among the various rays. Depending on the location of the earth and the season, ultraviolet light and all the other portions of light vary in intensity. This permits all life forms to go through constant cycles of change necessary for growth and renewal.

CHAPTER 2:
The Miraculous Healing Powers of Ultraviolet Light

Gone are the days when one's natural impulse was to step out of the house on the first sunny spring day to welcome and enjoy the bright, warm glory of the sun. Only the very courageous or downright 'careless' defy the grim warnings from medical mandarins and cancer specialists wholeheartedly endorsed by the sunscreen industry and dare to venture out into the dangerous sun. Some impractical practitioners of medicine consider it irresponsible and a 'potential risk' to walk out into the sun, if not fully geared for the onslaught of the hazardous sunlight. Unless covered from head to toe with sunscreen, people would be gambling with their lives, or so they are made to believe, by those who serve their own vested interests.

Sunlight is NOT life-threatening! It is in fact life-giving and life-preserving!

How otherwise, could mankind have ever evolved through the ages when sun block didn't exist?

Fortunately this absurd misconception is fading on account of the blatant absence of scientific proof that sunlight really causes disease. In fact, in contradiction, it is being discovered (or rather rediscovered) that lack of exposure to the sun is one of the greatest risk factors for disease.

For long now, the sun has been falsely accused of crime against humankind. The prosecutors, in majority, are the sunscreen industries and medical industry and we are the jury. It is only recently that we have begun to realize that there is no conclusive evidence against the sun. We are beginning to see that sun is, after all, not guilty.

Only the Ultraviolet part of the sunlight has been regarded malignant, but in truth, it has been found that UV radiation has a significantly vital effect on the human function.

So what is UV light?

UV radiation is one of the three different types of solar radiation. It is the part of the electromagnetic spectrum of light and energy from the sun that is invisible to the human eye and has the shortest wavelengths (300-380nm). Visible light and infra red heat waves are the other two types of solar radiation.

Although UV rays come naturally from the sun, there are also some manmade sources such as lamps and tools (welding tools, for instance) that can produce UV radiation. However, the sun is the primary source of UV.

Solar UV is never uniform in intensity throughout the day and in different parts of the world. It is at its highest at about midday. It has been estimated that about half of the total daytime UV radiation is received in the few hours around noontime. Apart from the position of the earth with respect to the sun, clouds and ozone also affect incident UV radiation.

Ozone mainly absorbs a great deal of UV radiation allowing only a small portion of it to reach the earth's surface.

Unfortunately, it is this attenuated ultraviolet radiation that is furthermore easily eliminated by windows, houses, spectacles, sunglasses, sun lotions, and clothing.

Windows under normal circumstances admit solar UV rays. But nowadays they are often installed with UV inhibiting films which are at the least 95% effective. Even prescription spectacles and contact lenses are made to screen UV radiation.

Before antibiotic drugs were discovered in the 1930s - penicillin having been the first one - before modernization met medicine, the healing power of sunlight was favored by the medical community, at least in Europe.

Sunlight therapy, called heliotherapy, was indeed considered to be the most successful treatment for infectious diseases from the late nineteenth to the mid-twentieth century. Heliotherapy fundamentally involves intentional

6

exposure to direct, natural sunlight. The objective is to avail of the therapeutic advantages of solar UV radiation.

Studies revealed that exposing patients to controlled amounts of sunlight dramatically lowered elevated blood pressure (up to 40 mm Hg drop), decreased cholesterol in the bloodstream, lowered abnormally high blood sugar in diabetics, and increased the number of white blood cells, which people need to help resist disease. Sunlight therapy even increases cardiac output and oxygen carrying capacity of the blood. Patients suffering from gout, rheumatoid arthritis, colitis, arteriosclerosis, anemia, cystitis, eczema, acne, psoriasis, herpes, lupus, sciatica, kidney problems, asthma, and even burns, have all received great benefits from the healing rays of the sun. Heliotherapy is even practiced in the Cancer Research Institute for successful DNA repair. It has been observed that cancer cells begin to die within hours of light treatments. The healthy tissue is retained and unharmed at the end of the procedure. 70 to 80% of the tumors treated have responded following only one treatment.

Sunlight is possibly the most powerful natural broad spectrum drug.

The medical doctor and author, Dr. Auguste Rollier, was the most famous heliotherapist of his day. At his peak, he operated 36 clinics with over 1,000 beds in Leysin, Switzerland. His clinics were situated 5,000 feet above sea level. The intensity of ultraviolet light increases by 4 percent for every 1000 feet of elevation above sea level.

So at 5000 feet, the sun's UV intensity is increased by a whole 20%.

The strategically placed clinics allowed his patients to catch a lot more UV light. Dr. Rollier used this UV light to treat diseases such as tuberculosis (TB), rickets, smallpox, lupus vulgaris (skin tuberculosis), and wounds.

He followed in the footsteps of the Danish physician Dr. Niels Finsen, who won the Nobel Prize in 1903 for his treatment of TB using ultraviolet light. In a span of 20 years, more than 2,000 cases of surgical (bone and joint)

7

tuberculosis were treated, and more than 80% were discharged as cured at Dr. Rollier's clinics.

Rollier found that sunbathing early in the morning, in conjunction with a nutritious diet, produced the best effects.

The patients (many of them children) were gradually exposed to the sun's rays until the whole body could be bared. In winter the whole day could be spent in the sunshine and dry, cold air. In summer however, exposure was limited to the morning hours only.

More than 100,000 lives were lost each year from tuberculosis, 'The White Plague' as it was then called. The miraculous complete cures of tuberculosis and many other diseases made headlines at that time.

What surprised the medical community most was the fact that the sun's healing rays remained ineffective if the patients wore sunglasses. [Sunglasses block out important rays of the light spectrum which the body requires for essential biological functions.] Note: your eyes receive these rays even if you are in the shade. By the year 1933, there were over 165 different diseases for which sunlight proved to be a beneficial treatment.

However, with the death of Rollier in 1954 and the growing dominance of the pharmaceutical industry, heliotherapy sadly fell into disuse. The gentle effectiveness of cure by sunlight was ignored and soon forgotten.

By the 1960s, manmade 'miracle drugs' had replaced the medical fraternity's fascination with the sun's healing powers. By the 1980s the public was increasingly bombarded with warnings about sun-bathing and the risks of skin cancer from exposure to sun. People were alarmed and even terrorized by the strong lobby of the sunscreen industry that put financial gains far above social health and wellbeing.

Today, the sun is considered the main culprit precipitating skin cancer, certain cataracts leading to blindness, and aging of the skin.

Only those who take the 'risk' of exposing themselves to sunlight find that the sun actually makes them feel better, provided they do not use sunscreens or burn their skin by way of overexposure.

While it is true that too much of a thing is not good, none of it is even worse.

It is true that overexposure to the sun can contribute to skin damage. But underexposure can be far more detrimental to health. We require optimal exposure to sunlight. A life of moderation in all aspects is a healthy one.

The use of antibiotics, which has practically replaced heliotherapy, has in recent years, led to the development of drug-resistant strains of bacteria, which defy any treatment other than the balanced use of sun, water, air, food and exercise.

Despite the remarkable advancements in medicine, the bacteria seem to remain a step ahead. You hear about some new promising drug and soon enough you are reading about a new deadly strain of some pathogen.

Cure only ensues when the body's essential requirements are in equilibrium.

Cutting out or substantially reducing any of the essential constituents of life results in disease. Disease is no more than a state of disequilibrium in physical, mental and spiritual function. Health will only be restored when the basic elements are well balanced.

The UV-rays in sunlight actually stimulate the thyroid gland to increase hormone production. Thyroid secretions largely control metabolism. Increased hormone production increases the body's basal metabolic rate. This assists both in weight loss and improved muscle development.

Farm animals fatten much faster when kept indoors, and so do people who stay out of the sun. Therefore, if you want to lose weight or increase your muscle tone, expose your body to the sun on a regular basis.

Any person who misses out on sunlight becomes weak and suffers mental and physical problems as a result. His vital energy diminishes in due time, which is reflected in his quality of life. The populations in Northern European countries like Norway and Finland, which experience months of darkness every year, have a higher incidence of irritability, fatigue, illness, insomnia, depression, alcoholism and suicide than those living in the sunny parts of the world. The skin cancer rates in these countries are higher, too. For example, the incidence of *melanoma* (skin cancer) on the Orkney and Shetland Isles, north of Scotland, is 10 times that of the Mediterranean islands.

UV light is known to activate an important skin hormone called *solitrol*. *Solitrol* influences our immune system and many of our body's regulatory centers, and, in conjunction with the pineal hormone *melatonin,* causes changes in mood and daily biological rhythms.

The hemoglobin in our red blood cells requires ultraviolet (UV) light to bind to the oxygen needed for all cellular functions. Lack of sunlight can, therefore, be held co-responsible for almost any kind of illness, including skin cancer and other forms of cancer. As you are about to find out, it may be highly detrimental to your health to miss out on sunlight.

CHAPTER 3:
Can UV-Radiation Prevent and Cure Skin Cancer?

Cancer is quite the modern day plague although it has existed for centuries. Studies now show that 25% of all deaths in the U.S. are caused by different types of cancers.

Cancer is a physical abnormality (called disease) characterized by the uncontrolled growth of a group of cells, which in most cases, results in the formation of a malignant tumor though some cancers like leukemia do not involve tumor formation.

The abnormal proliferation of cells is accompanied by invasion of the neighboring tissue in the body, a trait only exhibited by malignant or cancerous growths. Benign tumors are non invasive and so, less dangerous.

Another fierce feature that malignancies may display is metastasis which is believed to involve the spread of cancer to other distant sites/organs in the body, generally by means of lymph or blood.

Cancer arises from abnormalities in the genetic material within the cell. These abnormalities can be inherent or acquired as an effect of carcinogens or cancer-causing substances. There are many substances that have been found to possess carcinogenic properties but the most common include tobacco smoke, several chemicals, processed meats, naturally occurring toxins, irritants, certain radiations and viruses. Most of these are easily avoidable influences. More than a third of the cancer deaths around the world occur due to modifiable risk factors - cigarette smoking, alcoholism and unhealthy diets most commonly.

There are various types of cancers depending upon the site of the affection. The most common site in men is the prostate gland and in women, it is the breast tissue. But cancer can spring up just about anywhere in the body, including the skin.

Most skin cancers arise as a consequence of assault on melanocytes. They are often detected early because it is

11

mostly the outermost layer of skin or the epidermis which is visibly affected. Clinically, it is the most commonly diagnosed cancer. It is even more easily diagnosed than lung, breast and prostate cancers because of the obvious morphological presentation.

There are three main types of skin cancer - basal cell carcinoma (BCC), squamous cell carcinoma (SCC) and malignant melanoma. The basal and squamous cell carcinomas which are non-melanomas, are increasingly prevalent, whereas the third, malignant melanoma, is much rarer, but far more lethal.

BCC is the most common skin cancer. It is the least dangerous and does not have a tendency to spread. The usual appearance is that of a raised smooth pearly bump on the surface of the skin. If left untreated it burrows deeply into underlying tissue causing disfigurement and serious damage.

SCC is more dangerous than BCC as it can spread to other parts of the body. The clinical presentation of this cancer is most often a red thickened, scaling patch on the skin. These lesions are liable to ulceration and bleeding. If not managed, they threaten to develop into a large mass.

Cases of non-melanomas are more frequently reported than malignant melanomas. The majority of the people have BCC.

Malignant melanoma is the most dangerous type of skin cancer and has the poorest prognosis. It can spread rapidly. If not detected early, it is very difficult to treat. It accounts for 75% of all skin cancer deaths. This cancer generally begins in moles or areas of abnormal appearing skin involving the melanocytes of the outer layer of the skin. A change in size, shape, color or elevation of a mole may indicate a malignant melanoma. The appearance of a new mole during adulthood or new pain, itching, ulceration or bleeding is a few other signs that point to a probability of this disease.

Malignant melanoma has an affinity for Caucasians more than other races.

To be able to detect a malignant melanoma early, before it becomes incurable, one must carefully observe moles and the changes occurring in them if any. Some of the characteristic signs of malignant melanoma include

- Asymmetrical skin lesion.
- Border of the lesion is irregular.
- Color: melanomas usually have multiple colors.
- Diameter: moles greater than 6 mm are more likely to be melanomas than smaller moles.
- Enlarging: Enlarging or evolving moles.

Skin cancers have been linked with chronic inflammatory conditions of the skin.

Inflammations following overexposure to UV radiation and chronic long standing irritation of the skin (as may be seen in non-healing wounds and some viral infections) have been associated with skin cancer.

The non-melanomas are believed to be caused due to direct DNA damage provoked by UVB radiation. Malignant melanomas on the other hand are assumed to be caused by indirect DNA damage after exposure to radiation.[2]

Natural as well as artificial UV sources - sunlight and artificial tanning salons both have been associated with skin cancer.

Nearly 85% of skin cancers are believed to be caused by overexposure to sunlight.

In Canada, during the period from 1970 to 1986, the incidence of melanomas alarmingly rose by 6% per year for

---

[2] ULTRAVIOLET RADIATION is split into 3 categories- UVB and UVC, based on their wavelengths.
rays make up 90-95% of the ultraviolet light reaching the earth and have a relatively long wavelength (320-400 nm). These wavelengths are not absorbed by the ozone layer.
UVB rays have a medium wavelength (290-320 nm). They are only partially absorbed by the ozone layer.
UVC rays have the shortest wavelength (less than 290 nm) and are almost totally absorbed by the ozone layer.

men and by 4% per year for women. Australia had the highest melanoma rate in the world. For men the rate doubled between 1980 and 1987 and for women it increased by more than 50%. It is now estimated that by age 75 two out of three Australians will have been treated for some form of skin cancer. Recent studies surprisingly show that melanoma deaths are more in the UK than in Australia now. In UK there are 9,500 new cases of melanoma each year, and 2,300 deaths.

These studies are well documented and there is no doubt that skin cancers are becoming increasingly prevalent.

The most pressing question is why would the sun suddenly become so vicious and try to kill scores of people after thousands of years of harmlessness?

What revolution has the sun undergone in its behavior? Why is UV light suddenly such a taboo?

Before we begin to analyze this new found hostility, we must remember that the effect of the sun on human skin is influenced by three different factors:

1. The sun which is the very source of UV radiation
2. The earth and its atmosphere through which the UV waves travel (or get obstructed)
3. The human being whose skin receives the radiation

It is true that our skin is vulnerable to damage in the form of tans and sunburns. But to be able to make the connection between destruction of the skin to the extent of cancer and radiation, we must thoroughly study each of the three factors that control exposure to radiation.

Accordingly, the occurrence of skin cancer could be attributed to a change in the behavior of the sun, the atmosphere, or some change in us human beings.

There is no known striking rise in the amount of UV radiation leaving the sun. It is not the sun that has suddenly turned malicious and hazardous to humans.

If it is not the sun that has suffered any grave transformation in recent times, it has to be some change in either the earth's atmosphere or in our behavior that is altering our susceptibility to solar radiation.

The medical community has for long suggested that the dangerous alteration lies in the earth's atmosphere, ozone to be precise. They have pointed fingers at a changing environment and not at the individual human being. They are convinced that ultraviolet light is the ultimate cause of skin cancer. This theory is based on the assumption that the thinning of our protective ozone layer permits too much of the germicidal UV to penetrate to the surface of the earth causing destruction of all kinds, including damage to our skin and eye cells.

The theory, however, has major flaws and no scientific backing. Contrary to popular belief, there is no evidence that reduction in the ozone layer, as observed at the poles, has caused any increase in the melanoma incidence.

In reality, the germicidal frequency of UV is largely destroyed or is filtered out by the ozone layer in the Earth's stratosphere, so that only small amounts - necessary to purify the air we breathe and the water we drink - actually manage to reach the surface of the earth.

Let us further explore the baseless 'ozone depletion leads to skin cancer' claim. Several theories have been put forth linking ozone depletion to the skin cancer epidemic. Most of them revolve around the same basic model that -

1. CFCs[3] released into the atmosphere, over a period of time, infiltrate the stratosphere and release active chlorine. This chlorine destroys the ozone catalytically reducing ozone concentrations.

2. A thinned ozone layer leads to an increase in solar UV radiation incident on the earth's surface.

---

[3] CFCs are chlorofluorocarbons - the synthetic compounds of carbon hydrogen chlorine and fluorine. These compounds are used as refrigerants and aerosol propellants.

3. Exposure to more solar UV radiation results in a greater incidence of skin cancer.

These are no more than assumptions which have not been accurately authenticated and may well be erroneous.

To begin with, it has not been conclusively proven that CFCs are chiefly responsible for the thinning of the ozone layer. It is a topic of great debate.

While one group of researchers is convinced of the integral role CFCs play in ozone depletion, the other argues that CFC release has an insignificant effect on the ozone layer. This group believes that the natural sources of active chlorine easily surmount any contribution from CFCs, since volcanoes and the oceans discharge 10,000 times more chlorine into the atmosphere in the form of HCL and salt spray. The opposing group disregards this explanation and suggests that almost all of this chlorine dissolves in water droplets which never reaches the stratosphere and is soon rained out. CFCs, being less soluble, reach the stratosphere more readily.

Both of these arguments have their own deficiencies. Studies on different occasions in the past have corroborated both the opinions. Early airplane observations by NCAR scientists Mankin and Coffey showed an increasing trend of HCL caused by CFCs leading to active chlorine formation and ozone destruction. On the other hand Belgian scientist R. Zander published his results in 1987, showing no increasing trend in HCl. The apparent explanation was that natural sources of chlorine are predominant in the stratosphere. In 1991, when NASA researcher Curtis Rinsland and his colleagues found an increasing trend for HCl of 5 % per year, they concluded that both natural and man-made sources contribute.

Although in laboratories it has been demonstrated that chlorine readily destroys ozone, it does not happen so effortlessly in the ozone layer in the stratosphere.

Active chlorine alone can damage the ozone. But this chlorine generally exists in combined form as HCl. Hence, the ozone is not mercilessly subjected to the onslaught of a disturbingly large dose of this harmful chlorine.

What is the relationship between UV radiation and ozone depletion? Does a thinner ozone layer correspond to an increase in solar UV radiation reaching the earth's surface?

And is it of any importance?

First of all we need to know whether the ozone is truly depleting or not, before we start making claims about the hazards of the depletion.

Unfortunately there are certain limitations when it comes to measuring ozone concentrations.

For instance, studies by Belgian researchers Dirk De Muer and H. De Backer show that sulfur dioxide, a common air pollutant, can interfere with ozone measurements. This is so because both gases absorb UVB radiation in a similar manner. As a result, variations in atmospheric sulfur dioxide can be misinterpreted as changes in ozone. Thus, the decreasing trend of sulfur dioxide since the 1960s, in response to pollution control in the United States and Western Europe, simulates a 'fictitious' ozone trend.

The Antarctic ozone hole which is the temporary thinning of a portion of the ozone layer during the Antarctic spring in October is a genuine phenomenon. It is a transient phase that recurs annually. However it does not serve as a definite indication of a worldwide depletion in ozone.

A study of Punta Arenas, the largest South American city close to the Antarctic ozone hole, showed no increase in health problems related to depleted ozone. In fact, UV measures were too small to have any noticeable effect.

Ozone variations have a negligible effect on the intensity of UVB radiation compared to geographical variations on earth itself. UVB increases naturally by about 5000 percent between pole and equator, mostly because of the change in the average angle of the sun. Thus a 10 %

17

increase at mid-latitudes translates to having traveled just 60 miles towards the equator. Having said this, there is no reason for the man at the equator to be alarmed for the health of his skin. The greater intensity of UV at the equator does not make him more vulnerable or at a greater risk of acquiring skin cancer. In fact the incidence of skin cancer is much lesser at the equator than towards the poles.

The aim behind most attempts at ozone measurement is to monitor UVB radiations. Researchers have long labored to prove that UVB radiation on the earth's surface is increasing, to be able to corroborate with their global ozone depletion claim. However, they have been unable to yield evidence to support the theory.

In the past, studies kept conflicting with the supposition until a publication appeared in November 1993. A staggering increase in UVB radiation during the period from 1989 to 1993 over Toronto, Canada had been recorded. The new study seemed to finally offer a small quotient of authenticity to the grand ozone depletion theory. But after complete investigation it was found that the conclusion from the study was faulty. The researchers had unwittingly misinterpreted the short-lived rise in UVB radiation which was actually caused by a severe weather disturbance - the 'storm of the century' that hit the northeast in March 1993.

Although people are constantly made to believe that the amount of UV radiation is increasing steadily around the world, studies suggest the contrary.

Actual measurements taken in the United States since 1974 show that the amount of UV radiation reaching the surface of the earth is decreasing and continues to decrease slightly each successive year. This research was originally conducted with the intention of detecting the frequency of UV radiation that actually causes sunburn.

UV radiation had dropped an average of 0.7% per year over the period from 1974 to 1985 and continued to do so afterwards.

The fact that the number of skin cancers in the United States had doubled within this period of 11 years, completely contradicts the theory that increased UV radiation following ozone depletion is the reason behind the skin cancer epidemic.

Despite the many discrepancies in the theory that suggests ozone depletion increases skin cancer chances, people have nonetheless been driven to a state of panic.

The frenzy eventually led to the 1985 Vienna Convention which provided the framework for international restrictions on the production of ozone depleting substances.

Slaper et al. set out to assess the effect such restrictions would have on skin cancer rates. They conducted studies under three different circumstances.

One where there were no restrictions on production of the noxious substances. A second, which involved restriction on the production of five known ozone depleting agents by 50% and a third, where production of 21 chemicals of such nature was to be completely halted.

The studies were conducted presuming that the restrictions would be observed globally and that there would be no radical change in human behavior towards sun exposure. Based on these assumptions, the inference, in each of the three scenarios was as follows:

- Without restrictions, skin cancer incidence would quadruple by the year 2100
- Restrictions as observed in the second scenario would allow 'only' a doubling in the skin cancer incidence by the year 2100
- In the third scenario, skin cancer occurrence would only increase by 10 percent in the next 60 years

However the validity of these scary predictions was debatable.

The research was carried out assuming various rates of ozone depletion in each of the three scenarios through which

19

they attempted to estimate UV radiation levels reaching earth over the next 100 years. But one may question the worth of the entire exercise since ground stationed UV detectors do not even concur with satellite detectors.

Also, in their research, they assumed a dose-response relationship between UV radiation and skin cancer. It seemed logical to do so, the only hitch was that the studies were based on a dose-response relationship between UV and skin cancer in MICE!

The ozone depletion can cause no alteration in the incidence of malignant melanoma - which is the most disturbing form of skin cancer. This can be verified by the experiment conducted by Dr. Richard B. Setlow and colleagues at the Brookhaven National Laboratory, Long Island, New York.

The research was done on specially bred hybrid fish which were very sensitive to melanoma induction. These fish were divided into groups and exposed to and UVB radiation individually. The inference drawn was that 90 to 95% of melanoma induction was caused by UVA radiation. Since UVA radiation is unaffected and unabsorbed by ozone, the depletion theory can in no logical way be correlated to malignant melanomas. UVA passes right through ozone as if ozone did not exist at all. Even if all the ozone in the atmosphere were to disappear, the amount of UVA would remain constant. If malignant melanomas are triggered by excessive UVA radiation, ozone-depletion can in no way be held responsible.

Another point to be taken into consideration is that melanomas are more common in people whose work keeps them indoors for the most part of the day. Such an observation poignantly contests the validity of the declaration that increased UV light equals increased melanoma incidence. Another stark inconsistency lies in the fact that these cancerous lesions often appear on areas of the skin which are normally not exposed to the sun such as the eye, the rectum, vulva, vagina, mouth, respiratory tract, GI tract, and bladder.

The number of malignant skin cancers (melanomas) discovered in 1980 in the United States was 8,000 and eight years later it had increased by 350% to 28,000. In 1930, the expectancy of developing melanoma was as low as 1 in 1,300 people. Since 2003, 45,000 to 50,000 new cases are diagnosed every year in the United States.

Overall, since the beginning of the new millennium, each year one million Americans are being diagnosed with some form of skin cancer.

There are millions of sufferers now, all of whom have been made to believe that the depleting ozone has rendered sunlight dangerous. This has lead people to believe that the sun is the main culprit for their skin diseases. It is a sad and unfortunate and even harmful misconception.

Since UV radiation is actually decreasing every year and skin cancers were extremely rare 100 years ago when UV intensity was much higher and people spent much more time outdoors, what other factor could be held responsible for causing skin cancer?

If it is not the sun and not the earth that have turned hostile to life, the only other precipitating factor must lie in a changed behavior of man himself.

What could this change in man be?

We do know that is not a physiological or anatomical change. So, it has to be a change in our behavior, our actions.

As mentioned earlier, our skin is susceptible to damage from sunlight. But skin damage occurs only from overexposure to sunlight. There is a limit to which our skin can tolerate strong sunlight. Beyond that limit, our body signals out for respite. The obvious signs of sunburn appear. If we follow these signals and seek shelter, we eliminate chances of skin damage in a natural instinctive way. It is only by ignoring or suppressing these signals that we subject our skin to harm from overexposure.

Some of us consciously ignore the evident signs of sunburn on account of certain obligations. An appropriate example would be that of a farmer working in his fields or an athlete spending long hours on the tracks.

Yet others choose to suppress the innate indications of injury to the skin from overexposure to the sun by the use of certain suppressive applications. An apt example is that of a holiday-maker on the beach, sunbathing after applying an arbitrary amount of a sunscreen. This man in all probability may be unaware that the sunscreen is suppressive by nature.

Let us take the two examples of the ignorant farmer and the holiday-maker who is suppressing the body's normal response to overexposure. Both the farmer and the holiday-maker may be overexposed to sunlight to the same extent. Yet the holiday-maker who is suppressing his natural reaction, is at a greater risk of disease. This is because he is upsetting his physiology and not allowing his body to function the way it normally should. He is creating an unnatural condition for himself by applying sunscreen which his own body has not created and cannot recognize.

We are born with a natural sunscreen in the form of the pigment melanin. Any additional interference by the use of artificial sun-blocks totally unsettles the body's natural mechanism of coping with the overexposure to sunlight. The suppression gives wrong signals to the body which then fails to understand and reacts abnormally.

Our ancestors never applied sunscreen. What I am trying to reiterate is that, it is neither the sun nor the earth that is responsible for promoting the occurrence of skin cancer. It is man's changing lifestyle, his desire to find artificial substitutes that actually deprive him from leading a normal natural healthy life.

CHAPTER 4:
The More UV, the Less Cancer

We have established now, with proven studies that UV light reaching earth is not really increasing. But since a large percentage of the population worldwide has been misguided into believing otherwise, let us work out what the actual effect should be, of a hypothetical increase in UV radiation passing through our ozone.

Let us suppose UV penetration to the surface of the earth increases by 1% each year (which is not the case at all).

Even such slight increases would still be hundreds, if not thousands, of times less than the normal variations people would experience simply because of differences in geography.

Let us assume that you move from an area near either one of the Polar Regions, e.g. Iceland or Finland, toward the equator, e.g. Kenya or Uganda in East Africa. By the time you reach the equator, you will have increased your body's exposure to UV light by a whopping 5,000 percent!

If you live in England and decide to move to Northern Australia you will increase your exposure by 600 percent! Calculations show that for every six miles you move closer to the equator, you increase your exposure to UV light by 1 percent.

There is more sunlight and consequently more UV at the equator because the earth is a globe and the angle at which sunrays fall on its surface at different places is different.

The angle at which sunlight falls at the equator is nearly perpendicular to the earth's surface. However as we move away from the equator we find that the sunrays incident on the surface are at an oblique angle because of the earth's spherical form. The degree of the oblique angle gradually increases as we move closer to the poles.

As a result, the sunlight at the poles is much rarer than at the equator. In short, the UV at the poles is much lesser than at the equator.

Today, millions of people around the world travel from low UV exposure places to areas of high exposure near the equator - be it for business or for leisure. One day some place in Norway and the next day in Nairobi. Many thousands of tourists travel to areas that are located at much higher altitudes than where they normally live.

For every 100 feet of elevation there is a significant increase in UV radiation.

But this does not prevent people from climbing mountains or living in countries like Switzerland or at the high altitudes of the Himalayan Mountains. People travel from all over the world to these places just for the experience of a lifetime.

According to the UV/cancer theory, most Kenyan, Tibetan, or Swiss residents should be afflicted with skin cancer today. Yet this is not the case at all. The fact is that those who reside at high altitudes or near the equator where UV radiation is the most concentrated are virtually free of all cancers, and not just skin cancers!

This shows that UV radiation does not cause cancer; in fact, it can even prevent it. It is ultraviolet, not 'ultraviolent' radiation.

The human body has a unique ability to become accustomed to all kinds of variations in the environment. In other words human beings are capable of 'adaptation'. It is the process whereby an organism becomes better suited to its habitat. It is a characteristic that is vital to the survival of the organism.

That humans are phenomenal exponents of successful adaptation is obvious by the simple fact that while human settlements survive in the Sahara, Eskimos survive in their igloos too despite the absolute contrast in environment. Although human beings have broadly been classified under five different races based on their different geographical locations, these races are all able to interbreed: we still fall under the same species.

24

It is our adaptability has made us the most successful and dominant species on the planet. Our bodies show several kinds of adaptations to varying temperatures, pressures, humidity, sunlight, etc. For instance, humans show very characteristic thermal adaptations i.e. structural or physiological variations in the body depending on hot/cold environments.

Extreme cold favors short, round persons with short arms and legs, flat faces with fat pads over the sinuses, narrow noses, and a heavier-than-average layer of body fat. These adaptations provide minimum surface area in relation to body mass for minimum heat loss, minimum heat loss in the extremities (which allows manual dexterity during exposure to cold and guards against frostbite), and protection of the lungs and base of the brain against cold air in the nasal passages.

Moderate cold favors the tall, stocky individual with moderate body fat and a narrow nose, for similar reasons.

'Night' cold - often part of a desert environment, where inhabitants must be able to withstand hot, dry daytime conditions as well as cold at night, favors increased metabolic activity to warm the body during sleep.

In hot climates the problem is not in maintaining body heat but in dissipating it. Ordinarily the body rids itself of excess heat by sweating.

In conditions of humid heat, however, the humidity of the surrounding air prevents the evaporation of perspiration to some extent, and overheating may result. Hence, the heat-adapted person in humid climates is characteristically tall and thin, so that he has maximum surface area for heat radiation. He has little body fat; often a wide nose, since warming of the air in the nasal passages is not desirable; and usually dark skin, which shields him from excess solar radiation and may serve to lower his sweating threshold.

The desert-adapted person can sweat freely but must deal with the water loss involved; hence, he is usually thin but not tall. This adaptation minimizes both water needs and water loss. Skin pigmentation is moderate since extreme pigmentation is good protection from the sun but allows absorption of heat, which must be lost by sweating. Adaptation to night cold is also common in desert-adapted people.

The body is equipped with perfect self-regulating mechanisms that protect it against damage from the harshness of certain natural elements.

Overexposure to swimming in the sea or in a lake can lead to extensive skin swelling, shivering, and circulatory problems. Our body will let us know when it is time to get out of the water.

Getting too close to a fire will heat us up and encourage us to move away from it.

Rainwater is natural, but standing in the rain for too long can drain our immune system and make us susceptible to catching a cold.

Eating sustains our lives, but overeating can lead to obesity, diabetes, heart disease, and cancer.

Sleeping 'recharges our batteries' and revitalizes the body and mind, yet too much of it makes us sluggish, depressed, and ill.

Likewise, sunlight has healing properties unless we use it to burn holes into our skin. Why should any of these natural elements or processes cause us harm unless we abuse or overuse them?

Wouldn't it make more sense to say that a preference for unnatural things like junk food, stimulants, alcohol, drugs, medical intervention (unless it is for an emergency), as well as pollution, irregular sleeping and eating habits, stress, excessive greed for money and power, and the lack of contact with nature are more likely to cause such diseases as skin cancer and cataracts than the very natural phenomena that have ensured continued growth and evolution on the planet throughout the ages?

It is illogical to say that the same forces that have preserved life and provided for its propagation are the ones that threaten our lives today.

It is very encouraging to see that new treatments using light are increasingly being recognized as breakthrough methods for cancer and many other diseases. The U.S. Food and Drug Administration recently approved 'light therapy' to fight advanced esophageal cancer and early lung cancer - with fewer risks than are found with the use of surgery and chemotherapy. Although it has been known for over 100 years that light can kill diseased cells, it is only since a number of convincing research studies have been conducted that there has been a sudden resurgence of interest in light therapy.

There is promising success with bladder cancer, infertility-causing endometriosis, advanced lung and esophageal cancers, skin cancer, and diseases leading to blindness, psoriasis, and autoimmune disorders.

There is a new study that recommends UVB as protective to a total of 16 types of cancer, primarily epithelial cancers of the digestive and reproductive systems.

Six types of cancer (breast, colon, endometrial, esophageal, ovarian, and non-Hodgkin's lymphoma) were inversely correlated to solar UVB radiation and rural residence in combination. This result strongly suggests that living in an urban environment is associated with reduced UVB exposure compared to living in a rural environment.

Another 10 types of cancer including bladder, gallbladder, gastric, pancreatic, prostate, rectal and renal were inversely correlated with UVB but not urban residence. Ten types of cancer were significantly correlated with smoking, six types with alcohol, and seven types with Hispanic heritage. Poverty status was inversely correlated with seven types of cancer.

Scientists at Newcastle University have developed a cancer fighting technology which uses UV light to activate antibodies which very specifically attack tumors. They have

27

developed a procedure to cloak antibodies which can then be activated by UVA light and so can be targeted to a specific area of the body just by shining a probe at the relevant part. This procedure maximizes the destruction of the tumor while minimizing damage to healthy tissue.

The Newcastle University researchers demonstrate in the first paper the procedure of coating the surface of a protein, such as an antibody, with an organic oil which is photo-cleavable, a process called 'cloaking'. This prevents the antibody reacting within the body unless it is illuminated. When UVA light is shone onto the cloaked antibody, it is activated. The activated antibody binds to T-cells, the body's own defense system, triggering the T-cells to target the surrounding tissue.

When the cloaked antibodies are activated by light near a tumor, the tumor is killed. This work means that antibodies can be targeted to kill cancer tumors with much greater specificity giving fewer side effects.

These cloaked antibodies can be used alone, or in conjunction with the many antibodies already produced against a wide variety of cancers as bi-specific complexes. These complexes are formed from two antibodies, one antibody binds to a tumor marker, and the other with a T-cell. The T-cell binding end remains inactive until re-activated by light. This means when the bi-specific antibody binds to healthy tissues away from light, it cannot activate T-cells, resulting in far fewer side effects.

A study of rates of the disease in over 100 countries, published in the Journal of Epidemiology and Community Health suggests that lack of sunlight may increase the risk of lung cancer.

The researchers looked at the association between latitude, exposure to ultraviolet B (UVB) light, and rates of lung cancer according to age in 111 countries across several continents.

They took account of the amount of cloud cover and aerosol use, both of which absorb UVB light, and cigarette smoking, the primary cause of lung cancer. International databases, including those of the World Health Organization, and national health statistics were used.

Smoking was most strongly associated with lung cancer rates, accounting for between 75% and 85% of the cases.

But exposure to sunlight, especially UVB light, the principal source of vitamin D for the body, also seemed to have an impact.

The amount of UVB light increases with proximity to the equator as has been explained earlier in the chapter. The analyses showed that lung cancer rates were highest in those countries furthest away from the equator and lowest in those nearest.

Higher cloud cover and airborne aerosol levels were also associated with higher rates of the disease.

In men, the prevalence of smoking was associated with higher lung cancer rates, while greater exposure to UVB light was associated with lower rates.

Among women, cigarette smoking, total cloud cover, and airborne aerosols were associated with higher rates of lung cancer, while greater exposure to UVB light was associated with lower rates.

In one study, light therapy eliminated 79 percent of early lung cancers.

A similar study has been conducted determine a relationship between UV exposure and the occurrence of multiple sclerosis.

There is considerable variation in the occurrence of MS around the world which has been ascribed to environmental factors, like exposure to viruses or to genetic factors. One constant, though, is that prevalence rates are higher in places closer to the poles compared to places closer to the equator. For instance, in the United States the prevalence is about twice as high in North Dakota than in Florida.

In a recently published exploratory study, mortality from multiple sclerosis (MS) was found to be reduced by exposure to sunlight. Depending on the degree of sunlight exposure, the risk of death from MS was reduced by up to 76%.

Regular exposure to sunlight still seems to be one of the best measures one can take to prevent cancer, including cancers of the skin.

CHAPTER 5:
Now Even Doctors and Scientists Say: "It's Not True!"

Like myself, there have always been some health practitioners who didn't buy into the theory that the sun causes deadly diseases. It warms my heart to hear that now even some of the top authorities in the field are standing up for the truth, despite intense criticism from their colleagues.

Medical professionals are challenging the might of the meddling misguiding supposed 'doctors' who shamefully claim the sun to be the root of so many (manmade) evils and diseases. Doctors now openly say it is time we allow ourselves to benefit from the sun shine and not shun sunshine.

In an article written in the *New York Times* in August 2004, a high-profile dermatologist, Dr. Bernard Ackerman (a recent winner of the American Academy of Dermatology's prestigious, once-yearly Master Award), publicly questioned the commonly accepted assumption about the sunlight/melanoma link.

Ackerman was a longtime critic of the argument that sun exposure should be avoided, stating that the risk of wrinkles or squamous cell carcinoma from exposure to the sun needs to be balanced against the advantages from exposure to ultraviolet radiation.

According to Dr. Ackerman, who in 1999 founded the world's largest center for dermatopathology training, there is no proof whatsoever that sun exposure causes melanoma.

To substantiate his arguments, he cites a recently published article in the *Archives of Dermatology* concluding that no evidence exists supporting the notion that sunscreen prevents melanoma, a claim the mega-million dollar sunscreen industry and those in the medical mainstream have falsely made for decades.

The use of sunscreens became popularized in the 1960s. It was supposed to be a medical marvel in a bottle - the savior from skin cancer. The innumerable endless advertising campaigns have nearly given sunscreen a place (along with food, water, shelter and clothing) in the list of bare essentials for life. People are made to believe that sunscreen is as vital as the oxygen we breathe.

Unfortunately the general public seems to be unperturbed by the fact that the media keeps showing alarming statistics of increased skin cancer rates despite the popularity and widespread employment of sunscreen. Instead of questioning the efficacy of the sensational sun-block, the news of increased skin cancer incidence seems to be making people use more of it or at the most a different brand.

Among the researchers and professionals however, the ever increasing skin cancer rates are being acknowledged indeed, but what action is being taken in the direction is debatable.

Proponents of sunscreen believe that people stay in the sun too long without reapplying, and so they unknowingly increase their risk of getting skin cancer. Others point out that many people fail to apply the sunscreen in hidden areas such as behind the ears, thus increasing skin cancer risk with increased exposure.

Then there are those few who state that sunscreen has never been proven to prevent skin cancer and point to the lack of any controlled studies.

Although sun exposure is considered to be the noxious agent causing melanoma, it has been observed that melanoma occurs in areas where sunscreen is used the most and also that melanoma rates are highest among those that avoid the sun and work in indoor urban environments.

In August 1982 an article was published in the prestigious British Medical Journal *The Lancet* titled 'Malignant Melanoma and Exposure to Fluorescent Lighting at Work'. The authors of this study were the first to examine the possible relationship between indoor fluorescent lights and the ever rising rate of melanoma. Taking into account such factors as hair color, skin type and the history of sun exposure it was found that working under fluorescent lights had doubled the risk of melanoma in the subjects of the research.

In Australia and in England it was people that worked indoors that suffered from melanomas more than those that worked outdoors. The amount of UVB and emitted from these lights, the distance from the lights, how the light was encased, plus the wavelength of the fluorescent lights to the sun were compared. In addition, the use of oral contraceptives by women, were taken into account. Their findings revealed that most of the melanomas occurred on areas of the body least exposed to light such as the trunk and limbs (mostly the trunk in both males and females). They surmised that tanned skin from regular exposure to the sun actually protects the skin and that people who received more sunlight were less vulnerable to the deleterious effects of fluorescent lights.

Dr. Ackerman didn't stop at exposing the decades-long deception of the masses; he also cast doubt on the increase in the incidence of melanoma cases that medical mainstream doctors insist is happening. He found that an expansion of the diagnostic definition of 'melanoma' has allowed a much broader array of symptoms to be classified as the deadly disease compared to just 30 years ago.

Melanoma has to a large extent 'grown' to epidemic proportions because of statistical manipulations. In other words, if the same diagnostic definition applied 30 years ago were applied today, melanomas would have increased only insignificantly.

In fact in one of his papers, published in the *Archives of Dermatology* in 2008, titled 'An Inquiry Into the Nature of the Pigmented Lesion Above Franklin Delano Roosevelt's Left Eyebrow', Ackerman argued that the failure of Roosevelt's physicians to consider the possibility of melanoma shows the flaws in medical wisdom at the time for diagnosing such lesions.

Dr. Ackerman even challenged the medical mainstream to explain why nearly all cases of melanoma among certain races (blacks and Asians) occur in areas of the body that are almost never exposed to sunlight - places like the palms, soles of the feet, and mucous membranes. [4]Should it not raise doubts among physicians and patients alike when even among pale faces, the most common sites for melanoma (legs in women, torso in men) get significantly less sunlight exposure than other parts of the body?

Dr. Gordon Ainsleigh is a proponent of regular moderate sun exposure, which he believes can prevent a many as 30,000 cancer deaths in the United States yearly. A study published in CANCER (March 2002: 94:1867-75) bolsters his thesis. Rates of thirteen types of cancer were found to be higher in New England where there is a lack of sunlight in the wintertime. Deaths from cancers of the rectum, stomach, uterus, bladder and others were nearly double of that of people in the southwest. Dietary patterns were also compared and little difference was noted.

To make a point, based on this and other evidence, your best chance of avoiding melanoma is to move to areas of higher UV-concentration, such as mountainous regions or the equatorial tropics and become a nudist!

Since sunlight boosts the immune system, you may find that such a move would also help with many other health issues from which you may be suffering. Naturally, all this data raises the question, what actually causes skin cancer? The answer may surprise you greatly.

---

[4] Although melanoma has been rising among pale-skinned populations (who use sunscreens) worldwide, there has been no corresponding rise among native, dark-skinned populations, who have only one-tenth to one-third the incidence. Their skin's higher melanin level may protect them, but they also tend to spend much more time outdoors in normally higher concentrations of UV light.

CHAPTER 6:
Skin Cancer Caused By Sun Protection

The sun is completely harmless unless we expose our bodies to it for unduly long periods of time, especially between 10am and 3pm (during the summer). Overexposure to sunlight makes most people feel very hot and bothered and burns their skin. To avoid being burned and to find relief, our body's natural instinct urges us to look for a shady place or to take a cold shower.

This instinct is vital. It is by acting on this instinct that we preserve our health and keep our bodies from damage from overexposure to the sun.

When an irritating substance enters your throat (irrespective of whether you are conscious of it or not), your cough reflex immediately kicks in, so that your body can throw out the unwanted harmful substance. Imagine what would happen if your cough reflex was somehow suppressed. Your body would be unable to shield itself from the unnatural agent that would then more easily progress down the respiratory tract and lead to undesirable complications.

The cough reflex is an inbuilt and innate mechanism. Sunburns and tanning are no different. They are the body's reflex to undesirable overexposure to sunlight. If they are suppressed, the purpose is lost and the body is susceptible to severe damage from overexposure.

It is sad that the ordinary man is told: "The sun is dangerous! Protect yourself!" when what he should be told (if at all) is that the sun can be dangerous if you are overexposed to it and the only protection needed in such a case would be in the form of shelter, shade or clothing and not an application of something on the skin.

Sunscreen companies conveniently and unethically use the risk of skin cancer as the pretext to validate people's 'need' to use their products. They create a mass hysteria saying that sunlight is dangerous and people die from skin cancer because of that same sunlight.

If sunscreens are at all useful, then one must wonder how it is that there has been an exceptional rise in melanoma incidence in Queensland where the medical establishment has long and vigorously promoted the use of sunscreens. Queensland now has more incidences of melanoma per capita than any other place. Worldwide, the greatest rise in melanoma has been experienced in countries where chemical sunscreens have been heavily promoted!

Drs. Cedric and Frank Garland of the University of California are the foremost opponents of the use of chemical sunscreens. They point out that, although sunscreens do protect against sunburn, there is no scientific proof that they protect against melanoma or basal cell carcinoma in humans.

The Garland brothers strongly believe that the increased use of chemical sunscreens is the primary cause of the skin cancer epidemic. They emphasize that people using sunscreen tend to stay longer in the sun because they do not get sunburns, thereby developing a false sense of security.

Sunscreens usually block UV rays in two ways: either by using a physical sun filter, such as talc, titanium oxide or zinc oxide, or by using chemicals, whose active ingredients include *methoxycinnamate, p-amino benzoic acid, benzophenone* and other agents that absorb certain sun-burning UV frequencies while allowing others to pass through.

One of the oldest tried and tested methods in physical sun-screening is to use tin oxide as a 'reflecting' coating to the skin. Tin oxide is widely used in wound dressings and can be considered relatively safe. Applied as a cream it is visible in daylight. Although 'safe', there is a drawback as with every local application, it facilitates moisture loss. It should be avoided by people with dry skin conditions as it has a drying dehydrating action on the skin.

Many people will remember Calamine Lotion of old as both a sun protection and a soothing after sun. It has a Zinc

Oxide base. It is pink in color, visible in daylight and is easily washed off in water. It is likely that this lotion and some other 'reflective' applications are far safer than their colleagues, the 'absorbing' lotions which contain PABA and/or oxybenzone or benzophenone. But it is nevertheless a useless if not harmful exercise, applying these reflective sunblocks.

Let us divert our attention from these small-time criminal agents and talk about the real murderers - the absorbing variety of sunscreens.

Sunscreen with ingredients that absorb UVR can damage DNA when illuminated.

Some sunscreen ingredients generate free radicals and reactive oxygen species when exposed to UVA, which can increase carbonyl formation in albumin and damage DNA. It is also well-known that DNA alterations are necessary for cancer to occur.

Free radicals and reactive oxygen species cause indirect DNA damage in cells. Research indicates that the absorption of three sunscreen ingredients into the skin, combined with a 60-minute exposure to UV, leads to an increase of free radicals in the skin if applied in too little quantities and too infrequently, something that happens commonly.

What are free radicals and 'reactive oxygen species'?

Reactive oxygen species (ROS) are ions or very small molecules that include oxygen ions, free radicals, and peroxides, both inorganic and organic. They are highly reactive due to the presence of unpaired valence shell electrons. Reactive oxygen species form as a natural byproduct of the normal metabolism of oxygen and have important roles in cell signaling. However, during times of environmental stress (such as for example, UV or heat exposure) the reactive oxygen species levels can increase dramatically, which can result in significant damage to cell structures. This cumulates into a situation known as oxidative stress. They are also generated by exogenous sources such as ionizing radiation - UV for example.

Generally, harmful effects of reactive oxygen species on the cell are most often:

- Indirect damage of DNA
- Oxidations of polydesaturated fatty acids in lipids (lipid per oxidation)
- Oxidations of amino acids in proteins
- Oxidatively inactivate specific enzymes by oxidation of co-factors

What is this indirect DNA damage caused by free radicals and ROs and why is it bad? There are several types of damage that can occur in DNA. UV radiation is capable of causing two types direct and indirect DNA damage.

Direct DNA damage can occur when DNA directly absorbs UVB-photons. UVB light leads to a reaction within the molecular components of DNA in such a manner that there develops a disruption in the strand which reproductive enzymes cannot copy. It causes sunburn and it triggers the production of melanin.

Due to the excellent photochemical properties of DNA this nature-made molecule is damaged only by a tiny fraction of the absorbed photons. DNA transforms more than 99.9% of the photons into harmless heat. But the damage from the remaining < 0.1% of the photons is still enough to cause sunburn.

The transformation of excitation energy into harmless heat occurs via a photochemical process called internal conversion. In DNA this internal conversion is extremely fast - and therefore efficient. This ultrafast internal conversion is an extremely powerful photo-protection provided by single nucleotides.

The absorption spectrum of DNA shows a strong absorption for UVB-radiation and a much lower absorption for UVA-radiation. Since the action spectrum of sunburn is identical to the absorption spectrum of DNA, it is generally accepted that the direct DNA damages are the cause of sunburn. While the human body reacts to direct DNA damages with a painful warning signal, no such warning signal is generated from indirect DNA damage , and the indirect DNA damage is responsible for 92% of all melanoma cases.

Photo-protection is a group of mechanisms that nature has developed to minimize the damages that the human body suffers when exposed to UV radiation. These damages mostly occur in the skin, but the rest of the body (especially the testicles) can be affected by the oxidative stress that is produced by UV light.

Photo-protection of the human skin is achieved by extremely efficient internal conversion of DNA, proteins and melanin. As has been mentioned above, internal conversion is a photochemical process that converts the energy of the UV photon into small amounts of heat. This small amount of heat is harmless. If the energy of the UV photon were not transformed into heat, then it would lead to the generation of free radicals or other harmful reactive chemical species (e.g. singlet oxygen, or hydroxyl radical).

In DNA this photo-protective mechanism evolved four billion years ago at the dawn of life. The purpose of this extremely efficient photo-protective mechanism is to prevent direct DNA damage and indirect DNA damage. The ultrafast internal conversion of DNA reduces the excited state lifetime of DNA to only a few femtoseconds (10-15s) - this way the excited DNA has not enough time to react with other molecules.

For melanin this mechanism has developed later in the course of evolution. Melanin is such an efficient photo-protective substance that it dissipates more than 99.9% of the absorbed UV radiation as heat. This means that less than 0.1% of the excited melanin molecules will undergo harmful chemical reactions or produce free radicals.

The cosmetic industry claims that the UV filter acts as an 'artificial melanin'. But those artificial substances used in sunscreens do not efficiently dissipate the energy of the UV photon as heat. Instead these substances have a very long excited state lifetime.

This discrepancy between melanin and sunscreen ingredients is one of the reasons for the increased melanoma risk that can be found in sunscreen users compared to non-users.

A study by Hanson suggests sunscreen which penetrates into the skin and thereby amplifies the amount of free radicals and oxidative stress is one of the reasons for the increased melanoma rate.

The direct DNA damage is reduced by sunscreen. This prevents sunburn. When the sunscreen is at the surface of the skin it filters the UV-rays, which attenuates the intensity. Even when the sunscreen molecules have penetrated into the skin they protect against the direct DNA damage, because the UV-light is absorbed by the sunscreen and not by the DNA.

But what do sunscreens do about indirect DNA damage?

Indirect DNA damage occurs when a UV-photon is absorbed in the human skin by a chromophore that does not have the ability to convert the energy into harmless heat very quickly. Molecules which do not have this ability have a long lived excited state. This long lifetime leads to a high probability for reactions with other molecules - so called bimolecular reactions. Melanin and DNA have extremely short excited state lifetimes in the range of a few femtoseconds (10-15s). The excited state lifetime of these UV charged substances however, is 1,000 to 1,000,000 times longer than the lifetime of melanin and therefore they may cause damage to living cells which come into contact with them.

The molecule which originally absorbs the UV-photon is called a 'chromophore'. The bimolecular reactions can either occur between the excited chromophore and DNA, or between the excited chromophore and another species to produce free radicals and Reactive Oxygen Species. These reactive chemical species can reach DNA by diffusion and the bimolecular reaction will damage the DNA by oxidative stress. Importantly, indirect DNA damage does not result in any warning signal or pain in the human body.

The mutations which result from direct DNA damage and those which result from indirect DNA damage are different, and genetic analysis of melanomas can elucidate which DNA damage has caused each respective skin cancer. Studies using these techniques have found that 92% of all melanoma are caused by indirect DNA damage and only 8% of the melanomas are caused by direct DNA damage.

Direct DNA damage is confined to areas that can be reached by UVB light. In contrast, free radicals can travel through the body and affect other areas - possibly even inner organs. The traveling nature of the indirect DNA damage can be seen in the fact that the malignant melanoma can occur in places that are not directly illuminated by the sun - this is in contrast to basal-cell carcinoma and squamous cell carcinoma which commonly appear only on directly illuminated locations of the body.

Most chemical sunscreens contain from 2 to 5% of **benzophenone** or its derivatives (oxybenzone, benzophenone-3) as their active ingredient. Benzophenone is one of the most powerful free radical generators known to man. It is used in industrial processes to initiate chemical reactions and promote cross-linking. Benzophenone is activated by ultraviolet light. The absorbed energy breaks benzophenone's double bond to produce two free radical sites. The free radicals desperately look for a hydrogen atom to make them 'feel whole again'.

They may find this hydrogen atom among the other ingredients of the sunscreen, but it is conceivable that they could also find it on the surface of the skin and thereby initiate a chain reaction which could ultimately lead to melanoma and other skin cancers.

Kerry Hanson et al. have shown for the three sunscreen ingredients **octocrylene, octylmethoxycinnamate, and benzophenone-3** that after the sunscreen chemicals had time

41

to absorb into the skin the number of ROS and free radicals is higher for the sunscreen user than for the non-user. Such an increase in ROS might increase the chance of melanoma.

Sunscreen ingredients can also penetrate the skin. Between 1% and 10% of some sunscreen ingredients are absorbed into the body through the skin.

The absorption of the sunscreen ingredients into the skin does not occur instantaneously, but the sunscreen concentration in the deeper levels of the skin increases over time. For this reason the amount of time between the topical application of sunscreen and the end of the illumination period is an important parameter in experimental studies. Illumination of those sunscreen chromophores which have penetrated the stratum corneum amplifies the generation of ROS.

The Environmental Working Group (EWG), a Washington-based research group and habitual gadfly to the business world trashed any lotion containing harmful chemicals that can easily penetrate the skin. Oxybenzone, which blocks, is a main offender. The U.S. Centers for Disease Control and Prevention has found oxybenzone in the urine of just about everyone tested.

The British Medical Journal recently showed that sunbathers using some suntan lotions have a higher risk of developing malignant skin cancer, and a possible link with Oxybenzone. Oxybenzone is the chemical used in many sun products with high sun protection factors.

Oxybenzone's function is to 'filter' ultra violet light on the surface of the skin, converting it from light to heat, but it can also be absorbed through the skin. As yet we have not seen any research to indicate what happens when the oxybenzone is absorbed through the skin, but UV light causing cell damage is well known and readers may choose to avoid this form of sun protection. If light is converted to heat in the basal layers of the skin, damage to growing cells is very likely.

A recent report issued by the U.S. Food and Drug Administration included evidence that 14 out of 17 suntan lotions containing PABA may be carcinogenic, i.e. causing cancer.

Para-amino-benzoic acid works by absorbing UV rays in much the same way as oxybenzone. PABA, or para-amino benzoic acid, came on the market in the United States in the early 1970s and was the first true sunscreen to be generally available. They were the first ever widely marketed sunscreens.

PABA has the ability to successfully filter out ultraviolet rays from the sun. The advantage, that the chemical seemed to offer over others, was that it could stick tightly to cells in the epidermis keeping it from getting washed off in water or even rubbed off with a towel. The chemical is not used much in sunscreen formulations now because it frequently caused allergic reactions.

Through the years it was found to cause photo-allergic reactions to many people: a fair 1% to 4% of the population. As a result there has been a PABA sunscreen ban in many countries.

PABA causes DNA damage in human cells. Not only does it block out the healing effects of the sun, but it also promises genetic damage. Further research has shown that PABA causes increased genetic damage to the DNA in skin cells during exposure to sunlight. The damage done to the genes and chromosomes impairs the cell's ability to properly reproduce itself.

PABA was banned as a sunscreen ingredient several years after these findings were published. Phenylbenzimidazole (PBI) also causes DNA photo-damage when illuminated while in contact with bacteria or human keratinocytes.

Granted that UV light induces damage to the DNA in the presence of PABA, but to implicate UV light for this effect is tantamount to saying that oxygen is dangerous because when it reacts with carbon atoms it turns into a harmful waste product in our blood.

The only PABA ester approved by the FDA for use in the United States is Padimate O or octyl dimethyl PABA. This compound is chemically similar to PABA but isn't as irritating. Once PABA-free sunscreens were developed, the popularity of Padimate O declined quickly. Now Padimate O is used with other chemicals to increase the SPF of a product.

Researchers at the Harvard Medical School have recently discovered that **psoralen**, another ultraviolet light-activated free radical generator, is an extremely efficient carcinogen. They found that the rate of squamous cell carcinoma among patients with psoriasis, who had been repeatedly treated with light after a topical application of psoralen, was 83 times higher than among the general population.

For decades, government agencies and anticancer leagues have recommended the use of high sun protection factor sunscreens for the prevention of skin cancer. However, two recent European case-control studies failed to demonstrate any protective effect of sunscreen use against the risk of cutaneous melanoma. Actually, in these studies sunscreen use even appeared as a slight melanoma risk factor.

Careful analysis tended to demonstrate that the extra melanoma risk conveyed by the use of psoralen containing tanning activators is a direct one. Psoralens are medically used photo-sensitizers and potent tanning activators that have been introduced in Europe in some tanning lotions and sunscreens, either as bergamot oil or as purified 5-methoxypsoralen. However, following the demonstration of the photo-carcinogenic potential of 5-methoxypsoralen, it was questioned whether it was sensible to allow general population exposure to a carcinogenic agent for a purely cosmetic benefit. In countries such as Switzerland, a ban was imposed on psoralen-containing sunscreens as early as 1987, but was loosely enforced for several years. For more than 10 years, psoralen sunscreens remained the focus of debate. Developments of sunscreens combining 5-methoxypsoralen and UVB filters were followed by campaigns to convince the scientific community and regulatory authorities that these products were not only safe, but could even provide a better protection against sunlight than usual sunscreens, and hence were especially recommended to poor tanners seeking a suntan. Psoralen tanning lotions were authorized for general public use only in France, Belgium and Greece. In 1995, the first epidemiological study that examined the relationship between psoralen sunscreen use and melanoma was published, and demonstrated that poor tanners who ever used psoralens displayed a four-fold increase in melanoma risk when compared to poor tanners who used regular sunscreens.

In May 1995, the European Commission imposed a ban on suntan lotions containing more than 1 ppm psoralen (a concentration thought to be devoid of biological impact). However, this ban was effective from July 1st 1996, and due to the latency between the exposure to a risk factor and the onset of the disease, it is likely that the increase in melanoma risk linked to the use of psoralen containing tanning activators will persist for several years.

Sunscreens containing 5-methoxypsoralen (5-MOP) are being promoted commercially even now to increase sun tanning and sun protection. A recent study indicated that the 5-MOP concentration used in these sunscreens is too low to induce cutaneous photo-toxicity with ultraviolet (UV) radiation. An investigation was conducted to determine whether the sunscreen Sun System III (SS III), which contains 5-MOP, could induce skin erythema, edema, delayed pigmentation, and epidermal ornithine decarboxylase (ODC) activity when used in conjunction with radiation (320-400 nm). ODC induction is an early event in the promotion of skin tumors. Increased epidermal ODC activity has been reported after exposure to UVB radiation (290-320 nm) alone and with topical 8-methoxypsoralen (8-

45

MOP) plus radiation. Using a solar simulator, SS III-induced erythema, edema, and epidermal ODC activity were found in hairless mouse skin with only 5 joules/cm^2 of UVA. Human skin showed erythema and delayed pigmentation with SS III plus 20 joules/cm^2 of UVA. No photo-toxicity was seen in human skin unless the solar simulator output was filtered through water to reduce infrared radiation. This indicates that cutaneous phototoxic reactions to 5-MOP plus UVA are diminished by heat. Like 8-MOP, 5-MOP cross-links DNA and has the same skin photo-carcinogenic potential as 8-MOP. Therefore the use of phototoxic psoralens in over-the-counter sunscreens is inappropriate because of the risk of increased UV-induced skin cancer.

What is SPF? You may have come across the term Sun Protection Factor or SPF quite frequently. Let us discuss here what is implied by the term SPF.

With the exception of a very few, sunscreens are a combination of chemicals designed to protect the skin from UVB rays. SPF or sun protection factor is the ratio of the amount of UV it takes to produce redness or erythema on sunscreen applied skin. It is then compared to unprotected skin for 24 hours to see how much UV radiation it takes to have a similar effect. So if it takes 10 minutes for your skin to redden a bit, an SPF of, let's say 8, should allow you to stay in the sun eight times longer or eighty minutes before you start to redden. Chemical sunscreens primarily protect against UVB. In fact, if you were to take a look into the history of sunscreens you would be amused to learn that the first sunscreen to be formulated ever was known glacier cream and was created after a rather bad sunburn that the maker had the misfortune of acquiring while climbing a mountain in the Alps. Since sunburns are courtesy UVB radiation, an attempt was made at blocking out UVB without a thought cast beyond that. Goodbye UVB, goodbye sunburns. Unfortunately no one realized that it meant goodbye to good health too.

SPFs only apply to protection rating against UVB and NOT UVA.

In 1997, Europe, Canada, and Australia changed sunscreens to use three specific active sunscreen ingredients - avobenzone (also known as Parsol 1789), titanium dioxide, and zinc oxide - as the basis of sunscreens. In the U.S. the cosmetic companies have held off this policy as they try to sell off their stockpiles of cosmetics containing toxic sunscreens banned in other countries. However, avobenzone is a powerful free radical generator and also should have been banned. Avobenzone is easily absorbed through the epidermis and is still a chemical that absorbs ultraviolet radiation energy. Since it cannot destroy this energy, it has to convert the light energy into chemical energy, which is normally released as free radicals. While it blocks long-wave, it does not effectively block UVB or short-wave radiation, and is usually combined with other sunscreen chemicals to produce a 'broad-spectrum' product. In sunlight, avobenzone degrades and becomes ineffective within about an hour.

The simple rule of sunscreen - the higher the SPF and the thicker the slather, the better - has come under doubt.

The Environmental Working Group (EWG) has found that 4 out of 5 of the nearly 1,000 sunscreen lotions analyzed offer inadequate protection from the sun or contain harmful chemicals. The biggest offenders, the EWG said, are the industry leaders: Coppertone, Banana Boat and Neutrogena.

While 3 out of 3 industry leaders are rather upset with the EWG report, and while some dermatologists criticize it for hyperbole, the report does underscore several long-standing health concerns:

Sunscreens do not offer blanket protection from the sun and do little to prevent the most deadly form of skin cancer; reliance on them instead of, say, a hat and protective clothing, might be contributing to skin cancer, and the Food and Drug Administration has yet to issue any safety

47

standards, mysteriously sitting on a set of recommendations drafted 30 years ago.

As we now know, most sunscreens block only UVB. And the SPF system refers only to UVB. SPF provides an estimate of a lotion's level of sunburn protection. If you start burning in about 30 minutes, then SPF 15 will allow you to stay in the sun 15 times longer before getting burned - in theory that is.

In reality, the effectiveness of sunscreen usually wears off well before the calculated time and unsuspecting sunbathers keep applying very large amounts of these chemical poisons to their skin. The skin is not made of plastic, but of living cells. The constant biochemical warfare fought on the surface of the skin interferes with and destroys its own protective mechanisms, and makes it susceptible to permanent damage and abnormal cell growth. Such suspicions have caused some chemicals found in sun lotions, such as 5-methoxypsoralen, to be discontinued.

The main problem with using sunscreens is, however, that they may seduce sunbathers to stay in the sun much longer than it would normally be wise to do.

People fail to realize that near total UV protection is within reach and has been used for millennia. It's called clothing. There is nothing more effective than light well ventilated and yet protective clothes and hats when you want to spend long hours out in the sun.

The EWG report takes an axe to the loose SPF claims. Almost all sunscreen lotions contain chemicals that, perhaps counter-intuitively, break down in the presence of sunlight. But in fact this is how they block UVB from penetrating the skin, like a castle wall protecting against cannonballs until the wall crumbles.

Notions of all-day protection, as some sunscreen products claim, or even several hours of protection are ludicrous, the EWG said, because most sunscreens start deteriorating in as quickly as 15 minutes. This doesn't even account for sweat and casual rubbing, further reducing protection.

Also, few sun-worshipers use the recommended shot-glass-amount of lotion with each application. People readily think they are protected, but few really are.

A British medical report, released in July 1996 and published as the lead article in the prestigious British Medical Journal, showed that the use of sunscreens might indeed encourage skin cancer because they prompt people to stay in the sun far too long. Their use can postpone the onset of sunburn by many hours. Most people think that this is advantageous, whereas in fact, it puts their lives at risk.

The doctors who edited the report cited studies conducted in 1995 in Western Europe and Scandinavia that showed frequent users of sunscreen lotion actually suffered disproportionately higher rates of skin cancer. The report states: "Sunscreens containing only ultraviolet B blocks protect against sunburn and therefore enable greater exposure to ultraviolet A than would otherwise be possible to obtain." In other words, many sunbathers expose themselves to much more than they would if they didn't use screens. Sunburn, in fact, is the body's natural defense response against more serious damage, such as skin cancer.

Sunscreen is supposed to protect against two common forms of skin cancer, squamous cell carcinoma (SCC) and basal cell carcinoma (BCC). However, there is some evidence, largely arising from co-relational studies and in vitro experiments, that particular sunscreen ingredients (such as oxybenzone (also known as benzophenone), octocrylene, and octylmethoxycinnamate) are linked to increased risks of malignant melanoma. The broad areas of concern when it comes to use of sunscreen are:

- The potentially carcinogenic properties of some sunscreen ingredients
- Vitamin D deficiency caused by reduced exposure to ultraviolet light

- Incomplete protection against the full ultraviolet spectrum combined with increased time spent in the sun

These concerns have given birth to a sunscreen controversy within the academic community. It is known that some sunscreens only protect against UVB radiation, and not against the more dangerous spectrum. A number of class-action lawsuits allege that sunscreen manufacturers misled consumers into believing that these products provided full sun protection. The vitamin D hypothesis is not as widely accepted but continues to generate scholarly debate.

Chemical sunscreens are formulated to absorb UVB radiation. They let most of the rays through. Rays penetrate deeper into the skin and are strongly absorbed by the melanocytes which are involved both in melanin production (sun tanning) and in melanoma formation.

Sunlight contains ultraviolet radiation, largely in two forms: UVA and UVB. Aside from sunburn, UVB exposure causes the most common forms of skin cancer - basal cell carcinoma, which is rarely deadly and mostly only disfiguring, and squamous cell carcinoma, which can turn deadly about 1 % of the time.

UVA penetrates the skin more deeply and causes wrinkling eventually. Recent research, however, has found that it exacerbates the carcinogenic effects of UVB and may cause skin cancer itself.

Authors who claim that sunscreen use causes melanoma have speculated that this occurs by one of the following mechanisms:

- the absence of UVA filters combined with a longer exposure time of the sunscreen user
- less vitamin D generation in sunscreen users
- by reducing the exposure of the skin to UVB radiation, sunscreen suppresses the skin's production

of the natural photo-protectant, melanin, and the lack of melanin leads to an increased risk of melanoma
- free radical generation by sunscreen chemicals that have penetrated into the skin
- pathogenic cytotoxicity and carcinogenicity of micronized titanium or zinc oxide nanoparticles

Under normal circumstances when your body has not been tampered with by the use of sunscreens, your skin begins to itch uncomfortably when exposed to too much sun. In contrast, with the use of sunscreen you would not notice when your body has had enough sun because your first line of defense - unbearable sunburn - has been undermined.

Overexposure to, combined with external harmful chemicals and, perhaps, internal toxins, is the perfect recipe to damage skin cells and cause malignancies. Under normal conditions (without sunscreen), you would never get too much even if you lay in the sun for many hours. Although you would burn your skin through overexposure to UVB, you would still be protected against too much.

Some scientists believe that UV light causes skin cancer through the combined effect of suppression of the immune system and damage to DNA. Exposure to UV light is, however, not all bad. Dr. Ackerman discovered that although sunburn may temporarily impair immune functions and damage the skin, there is no proof that it can cause skin cancer. Most of the body's vitamin D supply, about 75% of it, is generated by the skin's exposure to UVB rays. Using a sunscreen drastically lowers the cutaneous production of vitamin D3. A low blood level of vitamin D is known to increase the risk for the development of breast and colon cancer and may also accelerate the growth of melanoma.

The British Medical Journal concluded that medical experts know "little about the precise relation between sunburn and skin cancer". This fact refers to all skin cancers, especially the fatal type of skin cancer - melanoma. Despite the colossal amount of research done on skin cancers, there

51

has been no indication that malignant melanoma has any links with UV exposure. But what is known for sure is that sunscreen not only fails to prevent skin cancer but, on the contrary, encourages it by amplifying absorption. This makes sunscreens far more dangerous than sunlight could ever be.

Dr. Gordon Ainsleigh in California believes that the use of sunscreens causes more cancer deaths than it prevents. He estimates that the 17% increase in breast cancer observed between 1991 and 1992 may be the result of the pervasive use of sunscreens over the past decade. Recent studies have also shown a higher rate of melanoma among men who regularly use sunscreens and a higher rate of basal cell carcinoma among women using sunscreens.

Dr. Ainsleigh estimates that 30,000 cancer deaths in the United States alone could be prevented each year if people would adopt a regimen of regular, moderate sun exposure.

Although the medical establishment still strongly supports the use of sunscreens, there is a growing consensus among progressive researchers that the use of sunscreens does not prevent skin cancer and, as a matter of fact, may promote skin cancers as well as colon and breast cancer.

In August 2007, the United States Food and Drug Administration tentatively concluded that "available evidence fails to show that sunscreen use alone prevents skin cancer".

Sunscreen ingredients are not tested in Europe, Japan or Australia for photo-carcinogenic effects before being introduced to the market. Even in the U.S., most sunscreens sold in 2008 have not passed regulatory testing either, due to a grandfather clause. Barely three new sunscreen active ingredients introduced in the U.S. since 1978 have managed to fulfill new testing requirements.

The use of sunscreen with a sun protection factor (SPF) of as low a value as 8 even inhibits more than 95% of vitamin D production in the skin. Recent studies showed that, following the successful 'Slip-Slop-Slap' health campaign encouraging Australians to cover up when exposed to sunlight to prevent skin cancer, an increased number of Australians and New Zealanders became vitamin D deficient. Ironically, there are indications that vitamin D deficiency may lead to skin cancer. To avoid vitamin D deficiency, vitamin supplements can be taken. Also, adequate amounts of vitamin D3 can be made in the skin after only 10 to 15 minutes of sun exposure at least 2 times per week of the face, arms, hands, or back without sunscreen. This applies in places where UV index is greater than 3, which is daily within the tropics and during the spring and summer seasons in temperate regions.

With sunscreen, the required exposure would be longer: if 95% of vitamin D production is inhibited, then it proceeds at only 5%, or $1/20^{th}$ the normal rate, and it would take 20 times as long - 200 to 300 minutes (3-1/3 to 5 hours), twice a week - of sun exposure to the face, arms, hands, or back for adequate Vitamin D to be made in the skin. Obviously, the required time would decrease with increased body exposure area, as when wearing a swimsuit on a beach, a very common setting where sunscreen is used.

By this math, it is apparent that vacationers who spend hours on the beach each day with sunscreen on may make more vitamin D in a week of vacation than they do during a typical week in their lives with no sunscreen, if they spend most of their non-vacationing time inside houses, offices, and other buildings where they get almost no sun exposure. Also, it is worth noting that with longer exposure to UVB rays, equilibrium is achieved in the skin and the vitamin simply degrades as fast as it is generated. It is thus clear that vitamin D overdose is nearly impossible from natural sources, including food sources.

The question remains: Can sunscreens that are made to block out both UVA and UVB radiation solve this problem? Research has shown that they don't prevent skin cancer either. First, the skin still has to deal with the acid assault that occurs when applying the lotion. Second, shutting out UVAs and UVBs deprives the body of the most important

53

rays of the sun responsible for maintaining proper immunity and numerous essential processes. The body requires UVB, for example, for the synthesis of vitamin D, without which we cannot survive. Is it surprising, then, to find that there are many people suffering from skin cancer today who have had either very little or no exposure to sunlight?

It is obvious that heavily-used chemical sunscreens are now being recognized as agents that actually increase cancers by virtue of their free radical generating properties. Some of these chemicals also, more insidiously, exhibit strong estrogenic actions that may cause serious problems in sexual development and adult sexual function, and may further increase cancer risks.

It is not that these compounds were ever viewed as benign substances. Organic chemists have been long aware of the dangers of compounds in chemical sunscreens. Such chemicals are widely used to start free radical reactions during chemical synthesis. These chemicals are the same dangerous types that one carefully keeps away from your skin while working in a laboratory. To be able to use them, chemists proceed to mix them into a combination of other chemicals. They then flash the mixture with an ultraviolet light. The ultraviolet absorbing chemicals then generate copious amounts of free radicals that initiate the desired chemical reactions.

We must realize that it is a dangerous thing to put faith in the hands of supposed health practitioners who deliberately promote and encourage the use of unnatural substances and activities. We have, for too long, been misled and suffered in darkness at the hands of 'men of science', when all along the power to preserve good health and heal ourselves has been within us. The secret is to reject unnatural things and elect to lead as natural a lifestyle as is possible.

We are in a constant process of reverse training our bodies to ignore the clues our bodies furnish when our heaths are compromised by depending on the doctor's declaration and modern medications.

We do not really need to rely on a word of another to decide what is right for our bodies and what is not.

After all in the past, medical professionals have let us down.

In 1927, 12,745 physicians endorsed smoking Lucky Strike cigarettes as a healthful activity. In the 1940s and 1950s, thousands of prominent surgeons were used in national cigarette advertisements to reassure the public about the safety of cigarette smoking.

In the 1950s, lobotomies were promoted for mental disorders and produced near-totally dysfunctional people.

In the 1960s and 1970s, diets high in omega-6 polyunsaturated fats and partially hydrogenated fatty acids such as safflower oil and margarine were recommended to reduce heart disease. However, long term studies found that while such diets decreased heart disease, they increased the total death rate and cancer rate, and produced accelerated aging.

Chemical sunscreens have three primary defects:

- They are powerful free radical generators. Their free radical generation increases cellular damage and changes that lead to cancer.
- They often have strong estrogenic activity. Estrogenic – 'Gender Bending' - chemicals interfere with normal sexual development engendering a host of secondary medical problems.
- They are synthetic chemicals that are alien to the human body and accumulate in body fat stores.

The human body is well adapted to de-toxify biologicals that it has been exposed to over tens of millions of years. But it has often had difficulty removing new and non-biological compounds such DDT, Dioxin, PCBs, and chemical sunscreens.

Why did this situation with sunscreens arise? Why was it only research scientists who repeatedly raised concerns about sunscreen safety? Why was the academic dermatology community silent?

Most of the academic community has a long tradition of informing the public about real and potential dangers to the wider social community.

Linus Pauling held a weekly protest in front of the Santa Barbara Library against the testing of nuclear weapons in the atmosphere. He continued his protests in spite of intense pressure from the U.S. Government and covert campaigns of slander against him. In 1952, the State Department refused to renew Pauling's passport. The official reason was that his travels "would not be in the best interest of the United States". Pauling was unable to attend a meeting of the Royal Society in London which was called to honor him and to discuss his ideas about potential structures of DNA. Many felt that he missed the chance to be the first to unravel the structure of DNA because he wasn't able to confer with colleagues. Although issued a short term passport in the summer of 1952, Pauling's requests for passport renewals were routinely denied during the next two years.

Pauling eventually won the 1962 Nobel Peace Prize for his campaign, and nuclear weapon testing in the atmosphere was terminated. But quite recently, a study by the Center for Disease Control estimated that the radioactive fallout from the atmospheric nuclear weapons tests caused about 11,000 deaths from cancer in the U.S. and produced a minimum of 22,000 new cancers. Some non-governmental groups are of the opinion that the deaths were far higher and nuclear testing is still responsible for 15,000 deaths yearly in the U.S.A.

Many other academics have, in recent years, led protests against actions and policies that were damaging to the wider community. These include campaigns to remove chemical toxins from foods, clothes, building materials and the wider environment.

This raises the questions as to why no member of the academic dermatology community, over the past 30 years, raised warnings about the dangers of chemical sunscreens. The answer is that the cosmetic industry has effectively silenced leading academic dermatologists by a widespread pattern of payments in the form of consulting fees, grants, retainers, vacation arrangements, and so on. In essence, industry has bought their silence on issues and products that might be embarrassing. Most academic dermatologists focus their attention on innocuous, safe, non-controversial topics that will not offend their corporate sponsors. They feel that the need to honor their agreements with their benefactors is far more important than the common you and I.

You must realize that big industries may not have your best interests at heart.

This may come as a rather rude shock to you but a Bayer subsidiary, Cutter Biological, was one of a number of companies that extracted clotting factors for treating hemophiliacs from pooled plasma. In 1992, the first cases of AIDS in hemophiliacs due to the medication appeared. The matter came to the attention of the Food and Drug Administration. The companies agreed to withdraw the product from the market which they did in the U.S.A. but not internationally. The administration went along with the companies in keeping the extent of the problem from the public. When they learned of the continuing international trading, they also remained silent.

Bayer had already paid for donors and for preparation of the products. It had US $4 million of concentrate in stock. In spite of their undertaking to withdraw the product, these companies did not stop selling internationally. Most countries in Europe read the literature and switched to the heated product. France was the only exception and those responsible were subsequently imprisoned for not acting responsibly.

Bayer and the other companies continued to sell to the East, to South America and probably other developing countries for at least a year. They even continued manufacturing the old product, possibly because it was cheaper to produce.

Bayer failed to adequately warn patients of the risks and played them down to its agents and to doctors. It asked them to use up stocks. Figures from Hong Kong and Singapore suggest that close to 50% of patients developed AIDS and many have died. Across the world it is likely that thousands were infected and died.

After learning something as morbid as that, it is not hard to lose faith in the medical profession. But you are not powerless. Nobody has to be a puppet in the hands of outright monsters. You can help yourself. You can live a natural, healthy life. It is only your decision.

CHAPTER 7:
Deficient Sunlight - A Death Trap

It has been known for several decades that those living mostly in the outdoors, at high altitudes, or near the equator have the lowest incidence of skin cancers. And as the evidence suggests, those who work under artificial lighting have the highest incidence of skin cancers.

We must understand that if we were meant to spend the greater part of our lives underground and hidden from the outdoors, only appearing socially at night, then nature would have arranged for us to be born rodents and not humans.

Fluorescent lighting may save money, but it takes a bigger toll on your health. The UV emissions from ceiling fixtures have been linked to a higher risk of melanoma skin cancer by the American Journal of Epidemiology.

Researcher Dr. Helen Shaw and her team conducted a melanoma study at the London School of Hygiene and Tropical Medicine, and at the Sydney Melanoma Clinic in Sydney Hospital. They found that office workers had twice the incidence of the deadly cancer as people who worked outdoors. The results of the study were published in 1982 by the British medical journal *Lancet.* Dr. Shaw proved that those who spent most of their time exposed to natural sunlight had by far the lowest risk of developing skin cancer. In sharp contrast to those living or working outdoors, office workers, who were exposed to artificial light during most of their working hours had the highest risk of developing melanomas. She also discovered that fluorescent lights cause mutations in cultures of animal cells. Dr. Shaw's research led to the conclusion that both in Australia and Great Britain, melanoma rates were high among professional and office workers and low in people working outdoors. In other words, the Australians and British (and the rest of us) would be better off spending more time outside where there is plenty of UV light! Similar controlled studies were conducted at the

New York University School of Medicine, which confirmed and substantiated Dr. Shaw's research results.

Fluorescent lighting has also been known to cause headaches, eye problems such as night blindness, fatigue, concentration difficulties and irritability. It has also been observed that an increase in the brightness of fluorescent light leads to higher stress levels by raising cortisol hormone levels.

In a study conducted on US Navy personnel between 1974 and 1984, researchers found a higher incidence of skin cancers among sailors who had indoor jobs than those working outside. Those working both indoors and outdoors showed the most protection, with a rate 24 % below the U.S. national average. Since none of the sailors spend their entire day outside, it could not be determined whether being outside all day would offer the highest degree of protection.

It is interesting to note that some of the hottest places in the U.S., such as Phoenix, Arizona, have the highest rates of skin cancers, but not because they expose their skin to the sun. Researchers are readily tempted to relate the alarming skin cancer rates to the sun and the fact that these areas are some of the hottest and sunniest in the country. But to hastily make that link without careful observation, without exhausting all possible parameters is foolish and irrational.

The extreme heat throughout much of the year keeps most people indoors during the day. As a result, although there is plenty of sunlight, people avoid it and develop health problems including cancers from underexposure rather than the other way round.

In addition, the dry hot air while outside, and the dry, cold conditioned air while inside the home, office building and car quickly removes any moisture from the skin, thereby leaving the skin with very little natural protection against the elements, fungi, and bacteria. Even during the night, because of constant air-conditioning, the skin is rarely able to breathe natural, moist air. The lack of moisture in the skin resulting from air conditioning greatly reduces its ability to remove harmful waste products from the connective tissues and other parts of the body. This can lead to increasingly weak and damaged skin cells. Unhealthy, irritable, dry, weak skin coupled with lack of exposure to sunlight and the poor immunity and vitality that result make the perfect ingredients for skin cancers.

It is a principle of physics that if you are in a dry environment, your body will lose moisture. Hydration is therefore very important and necessary to stop your skin from losing moisture and becoming dry. During summer, the temperatures usually increase and working in the hot environment becomes inconvenient. So we often resort to cooling the environment by the use of air conditioning or at least using fans to circulate air which helps to cool us off a little. In the case of fans, the circulating air helps to evaporate water (perspiration) off our skin and in so doing, the skin is cooled and this helps to cool the body. The loss of water through perspiration has a dehydrating effect on our skin unless we drink sufficient amounts of water and other re-hydrating fluids. Similarly, air conditioning moves/circulates air, which has the same effect as the fans, but in addition, an air conditioner removes a fair amount of water-vapor from the air while cooling the air at the same time, creating a much dryer, cooler environment in the air conditioned space.

Also, it is apparent that those who spend an inordinate amount of time in an air conditioned environment are not able to readily cope with hot summer temperatures. This increases reliance and dependence on technology and the resources it exhausts for unnecessary tasks, like driving somewhere within walking distance so that you don't have to face the heat.

When it is hot and humid outside and the air conditioner is not running, America suffers. Babies break out in rashes, couples bicker and even computers go haywire! In much of the nation, an August power outage is viewed not as an inconvenience but as a public health emergency.

In the 50 years since air conditioning hit the mass market, America has become so well-addicted that this dependence goes almost entirely unremarked. Air conditioning is built into our economy and our culture. Stepping from a torrid parking lot into a cool air conditioned lobby can provide a degree of instantaneous relief and physical pleasure experienced through few other legal means. But if the effect of air conditioning on a hot human being can be compared to that of a pain-relieving drug, its economic impact is more like that of an anabolic steroid. And withdrawal, when it comes, will be painful.

People are about as committed to air conditioning as they are to cars and computer chips. And a device lucky enough to become indispensable can demand and get whatever it needs to keep it running. For the air conditioner, that's a lot of energy!

Our absurd dependence on technologies like air conditioning and the unreasonable lifestyle compromises we make in response, contribute not only to the energy crisis but also to a public health crisis. Many people are made sick by extreme variances between outside and inside temperatures. Going from an outside temperature of over 100 degrees F to an inside one of less than 78 degrees is, for example, bound to play havoc with one's health. Severe heat waves are now taking a higher death toll than ever before.

Among the many disadvantages of circulated air from air conditioning units is the increased amount of mold spores floating throughout the house/room, as well as any sort of chemical by-products that get released into the air from appliances or cleaning supplies you may be using. Air conditioning keeps the harmful elements circulating, which can lead to aggravated sinus problems.

Air conditioners in cars also have their problems. Researchers at Louisiana State Medical Center identified 8 different types of mold living inside of 22 of 25 cars tested. Air conditioning units can also circulate air-borne diseases, most famously Legionnaire's Disease. If the unit has cheap filters or is not properly maintained, it will simply re-circulate pollutants.

Studies have shown that artificial light not only contributes to a higher skin cancer incidence but also prostate cancers in men and breast cancer in women.

Countries in which nighttime artificial lighting is used more intensively tend to have a higher risk of prostate cancer in men, concludes a new study that was carried out at the University of Haifa. This joins a previous finding that was published in *Chronobiology International* in 2008, that exposure to artificial lighting at night increases the incidence of breast cancer in women.

The study, carried out by Prof. Abraham Haim, Prof. Boris A. Portnov, and Itai Kloog of the University of Haifa, together with Prof. Richard Stevens of the University of Connecticut, USA, was intended to examine the influence of various factors - including the amount of artificial light at night - on the incidence of three types of cancer: prostate, lung, and of the large intestine, in men around the world.

Data was collected from a database of the International Agency for Research on Cancer, on the incidence of these types of cancer in men in 164 countries. Data on the levels of lighting at night were gathered from DMSP (Defense Meteorological Satellite Program) satellite images. The nighttime illumination data were adjusted by the geographic distribution of the population of the country, in order to reach an accurate measure of 'the amount of artificial light per night per person'. The researchers also examined additional factors, such as electricity consumption, percentage of urban population, socioeconomic status, and other variables.

At the very first stage of the study, it already became clear that there is a marked link between the incidence of prostate cancer and levels of nighttime artificial illumination and electricity consumption. Several different methods of statistical analysis were used to arrive at this conclusion.

Next the researchers isolated the 'amount of artificial light at night per person' variable in order to examine its particular effect. The countries were divided into three groups for this stage of the study: those with little exposure to lighting at night, those with medium exposure, and those with high exposure. The results demonstrated that the incidence of prostate cancer in those countries with low exposure was 66.77 prostate cancer patients to 100,000 inhabitants. An increase of 30% was found in those countries with medium exposure: 87.11 patients per 100,000 inhabitants. The countries with the highest level of exposure to artificial light at night demonstrated a jump of 80%: 157 patients per 100,000 inhabitants.

According to the researchers, there are a number of theories that could explain the increased incidence of prostate cancer due to exposure to lighting at night, such as suppression of melatonin production, suppression of the immune system, and an effect on the body's biological clock because of confusion between night and day. Whatever the cause, there is a definite link between the two. "This does not mean that we have to go back to the Middle Ages and turn the lights out on the country. What it means is that this link should be taken into account in planning the country's energy policies," the researchers pointed out.

The researchers added that an increased use of artificial lighting is considered by the World Health Organization as a source of environmental pollution. As such, the appeal made by Israel's Ministry of Environmental Protection to use energy-efficient lighting is problematic, as this type of lighting is also much brighter. The country ought to encourage energy saving in lighting as well as limiting the pollution level.

The average city-dwelling American spends 22 hours a day indoors, most of that time beneath and around artificial light.

Children, too, are increasingly spending less time outside in nature, and more of their time indoors at home, in school, on the computer, and in front of the television set.

During the winter season, most of the working population in the cities never even sees daylight, except through windows that reflect UV light. Incandescent light has a narrow band compared to sunlight, and exposure to it is known to weaken one's natural immunity. Our immunity is our defense against infection and disease. It is known that insufficient exposure to sunlight compromises our immunological function. Suppressed or compromised immunity means that your natural defense system against noxious entities is inefficient and insufficient. This further means that you are more susceptible to disease. A Russian study showed that workers who were exposed to UV light during working hours suffered 50% fewer colds. A weak immune system cannot properly defend itself against disease, and that includes skin cancer!

People with brown to black Afro-Caribbean skin and hair can spend long periods in the sun without burning. Due to their naturally darker skin pigmentation, African Americans are less likely than members of other racial and ethnic groups in the United States to develop skin cancer. They rarely suffer from skin cancer while living in their native lands where sunshine is plentiful. Their skins' high melanin level filters out a lot of UV but still provides them with enough of the beneficial rays. Although the rates of occurrence of various types of skin cancer are lower in African Americans, they are not zero. African Americans can develop skin cancer, and when they do, the outcome is often more serious than it is for other Americans. One reason why the outcome of skin cancer is often poorer in African Americans is that the disease is often diagnosed at a more advanced stage, when treatment is more difficult. Also, the type of melanoma most frequently found in African Americans is acral lentiginous melanoma, which is more dangerous than the types of melanoma that predominate in white Americans.

Statistics from various parts of the United States indicate that survival rates for African American patients diagnosed with melanoma are lower than those of white patients. For example, the California cancer registry reported a five-year survival rate of 70% for African American melanoma patients, as compared to 87% for white patients. Similarly, at the Washington Hospital Center in Washington, DC, the five-year survival rate for African American patients was 59%, compared to 85% in whites. The lower survival rate in African Americans was due largely to the fact that they tended to have more advanced disease - particularly disease that had spread to other parts of their bodies - when they were diagnosed with melanoma. When melanoma has spread to other parts of the body, it is highly lethal.

Among African Americans, melanomas occur mainly on body sites that are not pigmented, such as the palms of the hands, the soles of the feet, and the skin beneath the nails. Other sites at which melanomas occur relatively often in African Americans are the mucous membranes of the mouth, nasal passages, and genitals.

Like people of other heritages, African Americans should develop an awareness of the moles on their bodies and be alert for new or changing moles. In addition, they should examine their fingernails and toenails for suspicious changes, which may include brown or black colored stripes under the nail or a spot that extends beyond the edge of the nail. Anyone who notices such changes should see a doctor promptly because they may be signs of melanoma.

As has been mentioned above, people with darker complexions have lesser chances of developing skin cancer in their natural sunny habitats, which is why the skin cancer worry only truly comes into the picture once they move to more moderate or colder climates, like the UK or Sweden. Such a migration requires that they get extra exposure to the sun to maintain normal vitamin D levels since the sunlight in these places is far weaker than in their native lands.

In the U.S. 42% of African-American women of childbearing age are deficient in vitamin D. If the darker races do not get these extra amounts of sunlight, they are the ones who are most likely to develop skin cancer. The reason for their higher cancer risk is not *too much* sunlight, but *too little* of it.

As is so often the case, the purely symptom-oriented medical theories fall short in explaining the causes of disease. In fact, they are likely to make you ill. Beware of any advice given to you by any doctor, company, or organization who wants to protect you against a supposed threat while at the same time trying to sell you something else, such as sunscreen lotions. It is nothing more than a fictitious myth that sunscreen can prevent cancer. It would be unfortunate to get caught between the games played by the supposedly concerned cancer organizations and sunscreen industries. Keep in mind that when you pay for your sun-block, you are paying with your money and playing with your health. The outcome could be very grave.

CHAPTER 8:
Pittas - Watch Out!

Hippocrates was the first to write of the constitutional nature of the human organism. He taught that all diseases (excluding injuries) were initially general in nature and only become local to provoke a crisis at a later stage. All natural diseases are originally functional and then proceed toward pathological damage over time.

The old master also taught that there was no such thing as a single cause in a natural disease. He taught that causation was of an interdependent origin rather than any one isolated factor. There is always the merging of the susceptibility of an individual or group with a sympathetic pathogenic influence. Therefore, the etiological constellation includes the predispositions of the physical constitution and mental temperament, the nature of the disease state, as well as environment conditioning factors.

Disease is a state of disequilibrium in the mind, body and spirit. So as to understand disease, it is important to understand the individual before we consider a material cause.

According to Ayurveda, everyone is unique in their composition of both the physical body, as well as the more subtle realm of the mind, emotions and spirit. Ayurveda believes that our individuality comes from a unique combination of three basic operating principles, known as doshas. These principles can be found not only in our own human body, but also in every realm of the natural world. The doshas, or operating principals, are known as vata (ether and air), pitta (fire and water) and kapha (water and earth).

While all people have some of each dosha, most of us tend to have an abundance of one or a predominant combination of two.

The Pitta body type is described as-
- Medium physique, strong, well-built, medium height and slender. The chests are not as flat as those of vata

68

people and they show a medium prominence of veins and muscle tendons. The bones are not as prominent as in the vata individual. Muscle development is moderate.

- Complexion may be coppery, yellowish, reddish or fair. The skin is soft, warm and less wrinkled than vata skin. Freckles may be present. There is a tendency to easy sunburn.
- Uncomfortable in sun or hot weather; heat makes them very tired.
- The eyes may be gray, green or cooper-brown and sharp: the eyeballs will be of medium prominence.
- The nails are soft.
- The shape of the nose is sharp and the tip tends to be reddish.

Physiologically, these people have a strong metabolism, good digestion and resulting strong appetites. The person of pitta constitution usually takes large quantities of food and liquid. Pitta types have a natural craving for sweet, bitter and astringent tastes and enjoy cold drinks. Their sleep is of medium duration but uninterrupted. They produce a large volume of urine and the feces are yellowish, liquid, soft and plentiful. There is a tendency toward excessive perspiring. The body temperature may run slightly high and hands and feet will tend to be warm. Pitta people do not tolerate sunlight, heat or hard work well.

Australians who are not Aboriginals usually have fair and often freckled skin, reddish-blond hair, and light-colored eyes. Most Australians are *Pitta* types, which means that UV light penetrates deeper into their skin than among those who have darker skin or are *Vata* or *Kapha* types.

In addition, many Australians are fond of drinking beer, which has a strong diuretic effect and draws water from the skin, leaving it unprotected against heat rays. Both are risk factors for damaging skin cells.

The human body is composed of 75 % water and 25 % solid matter. To provide nourishment, eliminate waste and regulate all the functions in the body, we need water. Most modern societies, however, no longer stress the importance of drinking water as the most important 'nutrient' among all nutrients. Entire population groups are substituting water with tea, coffee, alcohol and other manufactured beverages. Many people do not realize that the natural thirst signal of the body is a sign that it requires pure, plain drinking water. Instead, they opt for other beverages in the belief that this would satisfy the body's water requirements. This is a false belief.

It is true that beverages such as tea, coffee, wine, beer, soft drinks and juices contain water but they also contain caffeine, alcohol, sugar, artificial sweeteners or other chemicals that act as strong dehydrators. The more you drink these beverages, the more dehydrated you become because the effects they create in the body are exactly opposite to the ones that are produced by water. Caffeine- containing beverages, for example, trigger stress responses that have strong diuretic effects (causing increased urination, at first). Beverages with added sugar drastically raise blood sugar levels, which uses up large quantities of cellular water, too. Regular consumption of such beverages results in chronic dehydration, which is a common factor in every toxicity crisis.

There is no practical or rational reason to treat an illness (toxicity crisis) with synthetic drugs or even with natural medications and methods unless the body's need for hydration has been met first. Drugs and other forms of medical intervention can be dangerous for the human physiology largely because of their dehydrating effects. Most patients today are suffering from 'thirst disease', a progressive state of dehydration in certain areas of the body. Unable to remove toxins from these parts due to insufficient water supply, the body is faced with the consequences of their destructive effects. The lack of recognition of the most basic aspects of water metabolism in our body can be held responsible for seeing a disease when it really is the body's urgent cry for water.

The *melanocyte* cells of our skin release *melanin* when exposed to sunlight. *Melanin* is the skin's protective darkening pigment whose presence we refer to as a tan. Pitta types are very sensitive to heat, and their bodies will quickly tell them if the amount of *melanin* produced is not sufficient to protect them against burning.

Pitta types should, therefore, *not* use sunscreens. Blocking out UVB may be disastrous for their skin. Blocking out both UVB and UVA all together can undermine proper vitamin D synthesis and upset some of the most basic functions in their body.

The adverse effect of sunscreen on such people is something equivalent to getting a muscle pull for which a painkiller is taken. Though the painkiller successfully reduces the pain, it has no therapeutic effect for the primary clinical condition - the pull. Instead the painkiller gives the person a false feeling that the problem is solved. He then engages in manual/physical work when he actually should be giving the muscle complete rest so that it heals. The point is that the damage is continuing unchecked and unnoticed as it is masked by the action of the pain reliever.

It should also be borne in mind that the Pitta types are also the first to react to the presence of harmful chemicals and poisons, developing multiple chemical sensitivities and allergies.

If Pittas expose themselves to the direct sun (avoiding the sun from 10:00 a.m. to 3:00 p.m.) for just a few minutes a day, they will soon be able to increase their body's exposure to a maximum of 20 minutes a day without having any signs of reddening. The process is gradual and most rewarding. Their skin will improve and *melanin* production will increase. This exposure to the sun will give them enough UV light to remain healthy, provided they do **not** use devices and solutions that alter or filter out light, including

71

sunscreens or sunglasses. Exposing their skin to the sun under the influence of alcohol or other diuretics, such as coffee, tea, and soft drinks greatly increases the chance of damaging the skin.

CHAPTER 9:
No Sun, No Health!

A balanced diet of sunlight, which varies according to body type and racial color, includes all the various frequency bands of ultraviolet light reaching the earth. Along with nutritious food and a balanced lifestyle, sunlight still offers the best protection against all types of diseases. Solar research from all over the world has shown that exposure to ultraviolet light is probably the most comprehensive and impressive healing method there is.

With all of the tremendous benefits that sunlight has been proven to bestow upon us, it is truly astonishing that most of the sick people in the world still rely on expensive and poisonous medical drugs that do not offer nearly as many benefits.

Modern medicine has become dangerous because many use it for selfish purposes and to profit out of people's illnesses. It is a known fact that medical workers and physicians engage in cut-practices or fee-sharing to exploit patients. There are innumerable medicines sold in the market which are completely unnecessary and worthless. Doctors prescribe costly medicines to get commission. It is well known that 60% of kidney failures are due to the use of drugs. Many painkillers are cancer inducing. Many medicines have side effects, short term and long term, and in some cases lasting throughout life. For a simple viral fever and common cold there is no specific effective medicine. Use of powerful and vague medicines decrease natural immunity and the condition of the patient, is only likely to worsen. The use of cortisones and other medicines is known to decrease immunity in asthma patients. There is again no definite medicine in allopathy for the treatment of common jaundice.

Despite the obvious hazards of modern medicines, the very fact that they are so successful in the market only proves that people are being thoroughly deceived by the people they should trust the most - their doctors.

It is time to step into the age of awareness and realize how harmful it is to resort to the most unnatural means of relief from disease. It is far better to remember and benefit from the natural healthy, gentle, life-saving remedies in our environment. The best things in nature come free. There is plenty of sunlight. We have only our health to preserve through is appropriate use, and useful it is indeed!

The following are a few examples of what ultraviolet light from the sun can do for you:

Ultraviolet light
- Improves electrocardiogram readings
- Lowers blood pressure and resting heart rate
- Improves cardiac output
- Reduces cholesterol, if required
- Increases glycogen stores in the liver
- Balances blood sugar
- Enhances energy, endurance, and muscular strength
- Improves the body's resistance to infections due to an increase of lymphocytes and phagocytic index (the average number of bacteria ingested per leukocyte of the patient's blood)
- Enhances the oxygen-carrying capacity of the blood
- Increases sex hormones
- Improves resistance of the skin to infections
- Raises one's tolerance to stress and reduces depression

Sunlight not only purifies seawater to a depth of 12 feet, but it also disinfects the skin from harmful germs.

Ultraviolet germicidal irradiation or (UVGI) is a sterilization method that uses ultraviolet (UV) light to break down microorganisms. This form of UV radiation is industrially used to purify and sterilize food, water, air and instruments. UVGI utilizes the short wavelength of UV that is harmful to forms of life at the micro-organic level. It is effective in destroying the nucleic acids in these organisms so that their DNA is disrupted by the UV radiation. This removes their reproductive capabilities and kills them. The wavelength of UV that causes this effect is rare on Earth as its atmosphere blocks it. Using a UVGI device in certain environments like circulating air or water systems creates a deadly effect on micro-organisms such as pathogens, viruses and molds that are in these environments. Coupled with a filtration system, UVGI can remove harmful micro-organisms from these environments.

There are no micro-organisms known to be resistant to UV, unlike chlorination. UV is known to be highly effective against bacteria, viruses, algae, molds and yeasts, and disease causing oocysts like cryptosporidium and giardia. In practice, bacteria and viruses are the cause of most major waterborne pathogenic diseases. Of these enteric viruses, hepatitis virus and Legionella pneumophila have been shown to survive for considerable periods in the presence of chlorine, but are readily eliminated by UV treatment. For most microorganisms, the removal efficiency of UV for microbiological contaminants such as bacteria and virus generally exceeds 99.99%. Specifically, the following are moved to an efficiency of greater than 99.99%: E-coli, Salmonella typhi (Typhoid fever), Salmonella enteritidis (Gastroenteritis), Vibrio cholerae (Cholera), Mycobacetrium Tuberculosis (Tuberculosis), Legionella pneumophila (Legionnaires' Disease), Influenza Virus, Polio virus, and Hepatitis A Virus (better than 90%).

The longer the ultraviolet wavelength, the deeper it penetrates the skin. At 290nm (one nanometer or nm equals one billionth of a meter), about 50% of the ultraviolet light penetrates a little deeper than to the superficial layers of the skin, whereas at 400nm, 50% reaches the deeper layers. The deeper-reaching rays can even penetrate the brain.

The human body was designed to absorb UV light for very good reasons; otherwise we would have been born with a natural absolute sunscreen for UV light on our skin and in our eyes. One of the most important reasons is that UV radiation is necessary for normal cell division. A lack of UV light disturbs normal cell growth, which can lead to cancer, as confirmed by Dr. Shaw's research.

The use of sunglasses, including regular UV reflecting spectacles and contact lenses are co-responsible for certain degenerative eye diseases, such as macular degeneration.

Most people who use sunglasses report continuously weakening eyesight. The solution is to this problem is simple: stop wearing them or begin to phase out your sunglasses. You will soon discover that your eyes are gradually getting used to sunlight again.

There are other ways to improve eyesight and reduce sensitivity to sunlight. These primarily include eye-exercises, good nutrition (consisting of mostly alkaline-forming foods), and avoiding eyestrain and watching too many hours of television.

Our typical indoor lifestyle, coupled with excessive over-stimulation through highly acid-forming foods and beverages, the cholesterol-increasing and dehydrating effects of television, and various other stress factors are sufficient cause for damage to body cells, including those that make up the eyes.

The Sun is important for our eye-health. Sunshine enables us to manufacture the Vitamin D that we need. Eyes that have been deprived of sunshine are pale and lifeless. Extreme sensitivity to sunshine is called photophobia. People who are sensitive to light and glare usually solve their problem by wearing sunglasses. But is that a solution or a stop-gap measure?

Sunglasses prevent our eyes from getting adequate sunlight and causes even greater light sensitivity. The more we wear them, the more we are sensitive to light. Hence a vicious cycle develops!

By sunning our eyes, we can reduce our sensitivity to light and sharpen our eyesight. Many people have reported that their vision improved after sunning - a simple eye exercise. Sunning must be ideally done in the morning or evening and never during the hot afternoon sun. Do a moderate amount for each session. There is no need to sun your eyes until you are sun burnt. The procedure is simple. Close your eyes and face the sun directly. Slowly move your head to the left and then to the right to let the sunshine reach every part of your retina.

By regularly shutting out much-needed UV light (even children and some pets are given sunglasses to wear nowadays), the eyes are unable to properly repair themselves and replace worn out eye cells.

The increased incidence of blindness and eye diseases in the industrialized world may result, to a large extent, from the misinformation that the sun is dangerous. Please be aware that in sunny parts of the world, almost everyone wears sunglasses nowadays. This may very well account for the increase of cataracts in these places. There may also be other factors involved, such as malnutrition (diarrhea can lead to severe demineralization), smoking, pollution, and poor diet. It is known that disease is not caused by a single reason alone. It is the cumulative effect of morbid environmental agents and also our habits and practices - dietary, behavioral, etc. To keep your eyes healthy, be sure to allow enough direct or indirect sunlight to enter your eyes, ideally no less than one hour every day.

The reason so many people are attracted to being in the sun or long for it when it doesn't shine is inherent in the natural instinct of the body to expose itself to the healing and cleansing properties of sunlight. The body is more intelligent than we give it credit for. While we believe that the mind governs the body, we must not forget that the body just as well affects the mind. The two function jointly in synchronization as a unit and must not be resolved into two individual elements. We must respect our innate corporeal intelligence. Without being tricked into overexposure by 'protective' sunscreens, the body will naturally know how much sunlight is good for its balanced growth. And even if circumstances lead to sunburn, the human body is perfectly equipped to handle that. Chemical interference in this process of self-protection, however, can have serious consequences.

By regularly using any of the following drugs or chemicals internally or externally, both skin and eyes become oversensitive to sunlight, and the skin may badly burn, even after a few minutes of exposure.

Among these are antibacterial agents such as Sulfa, the aforementioned PABAs and other sun lotion ingredients, hypoglycemic agents used by diabetics, diuretics for control of high blood pressure, tranquillizers and anti-depressants, broad-spectrum antibiotics, anti-arrhythmic Quinidine used to suppress abnormal heart rhythms, halogenated, antiseptic compounds used in cosmetics, many types of soaps, synthetic ingredients in most commercial beauty products, and antihistamines used for colds and allergies.

In addition, gallstones in the liver prevent the liver from sufficiently detoxifying pharmaceutical drugs, alcohol, and other noxious substances. There are over 1,000 drugs and chemicals that are capable of causing injury to the liver. The terms drug-induced liver disease, drug hepatotoxicity, and drug-induced hepatitis are used to describe those instances in which a medication or chemical substance has caused injury to the liver. Drug-induced liver injury may account for as many as 10 % of hepatitis cases in adults overall, 40 % of hepatitis cases in adults over fifty years old, and 25 % of cases of fulminant liver failure.

There is a rigorous process - known as clinical trials, that a drug must go through before it is determined to be safe for the public. These clinical trials are conducted on a carefully selected group of people who have met a long list of criteria in order to be able to participate in the testing of the medication. However, after the FDA has approved a particular drug, a larger and more varied group of people will be taking the drug. This more diverse group of people may have additional medical problems that were not encountered during the testing of the medication. This is why occasionally, a drug originally thought to be safe, may be discovered to cause severe liver injury. In fact, drug-induced liver injury is the most common reason for the withdrawal from the market of an already FDA approved drug. Two examples of drugs withdrawn from the market due to severe liver injury include Duract (bromfenac), a nonsteroidal anti-inflammatory medication, and Rezulin (troglitasone) a diabetic medication.

Since all medications are processed through the liver at least to some degree, people with liver disease must become aware of which medications can cause liver damage, which medications can worsen pre-existing liver disease, and which medications are safe to take. It is the liver's job to detoxify any substances that are potentially harmful to the body. An already damaged and weakened liver must work much harder than a healthy liver in order to accomplish this task. When a person with liver disease ingests a potentially hepatotoxic drug, this puts an additional strain on the liver and can result in further liver injury or possibly even liver failure. Even people with a healthy liver can develop liver disease as a consequence of ingesting a toxic medication or drug.

A particular drug may cause liver damage for many reasons. First, there are some drugs that are intrinsically toxic to the liver. These drugs can cause liver injury when the drug is taken in a dosage that exceeds the recommended dosage. This form of drug hepatotoxicity is what is known as 'dose-dependent'.

The greater the amount by which the dosage taken exceeds the recommended dose, the more likely it is that the drug will cause liver injury. Drugs in this category are usually broken down by the cytochrome P450 enzyme system. Under normal circumstances, the cytochrome P450 enzyme system usually converts toxic substances into nontoxic ones. However, in situations of drug hepatotoxicity, the reverse happens. A non-hepatotoxic drug is broken down into hepatotoxic byproducts. These byproducts cause liver damage as they begin to accumulate. An example of a drug in this category is the headache and minor pain reliever acetaminophen (Tylenol). The drugs in this category may also cause liver injury if taken in excess in combination with another hepatotoxic substance, such as alcohol.

Second, there are some drugs that can trigger an idiosyncratic reaction (an abnormal, unexpected hypersensitivity) to a normal dose of the drug similar to an allergic reaction, even though a normal dose may have been taken. Such a reaction is not related to the quantity of the drug ingested, and furthermore, the ensuing liver injury is unpredictable. This type of drug hepatotoxicity is often accompanied by fatigue, fever, and rash. It usually develops after a person has already been taking the drug for a few weeks. An example of a drug in this category is the anticonvulsant phenytoin (Dilantin).

Finally, a person's susceptibility to a potentially hepatotoxic drug is enhanced by many factors. Some of these factors are within the person's control, such as cigarette smoking and excessive alcohol intake. But other factors cannot be altered. These include advancing age and being of the female gender. Many of the relevant factors, both alterable as well as permanent, are listed below.

- Age. Adults are more prone to liver injury from certain hepatotoxic drugs such as isoniazide (INH), a drug used to treat tuberculosis.
- Gender. Females are more susceptible than males are to most forms of drug-induced liver disease - especially drugs that can cause chronic hepatitis, such as methyldopa (Aldomet) - a drug used to treat hypertension (high blood pressure).

- Genetics. Some people have a genetically based impaired ability to break down potentially hepatotoxic drugs into safe byproducts, such as phenytoin (Dilantin) - a drug used to treat seizures.
- Dose. The higher the dose, the greater the risk of liver toxicity. This applies to drugs such as acetaminophen (Tylenol), which are by nature potentially toxic to the liver.
- Duration. For some drugs such as methotrexate (a type of chemotherapy), the longer it is used, the greater the likelihood of liver damage or even cirrhosis.
- Kidney damage. People with poorly functioning kidneys are more prone to the hepatotoxicity of some drugs such as tetracycline - an antibiotic.
- Alcohol. Alcohol consumption enhances the hepatotoxicity of certain drugs, such as acetaminophen.
- Cigarettes. Cigarette smoking enhances the hepatotoxicity of certain drugs, such as acetaminophen.
- Drug interactions. Taking two hepatotoxic drugs in combination can greatly increase the likelihood of liver damage compared with taking one hepatotoxic drug alone.
- Hepatitis C. The presence of hepatitis C may increase the hepatotoxic potential of certain drugs such as the non-steroidal anti-inflammatory (NSAID) ibuprofen (Motrin), and certain medications used in the treatment of HIV.
- HIV. The presence of HIV (the virus which causes AIDS) increases the likelihood of hepatotoxicity from certain drugs such as sulfamethoxazole-trimethoprim (Septra).
- Rheumatoid arthritis (RA) and systemic lupus erythematosus (SLE). People with these autoimmune

disorders are more prone to the hepatotoxic effects of aspirin than people without these disorders.

- Obesity. Obesity increases the susceptibility of halothane-induced liver injury. (Halothane is a type of anesthesia.)
- Nutritional status. Either fasting or a high protein diet can increase a person's susceptibility to acetaminophen-induced liver injury.

Whatever toxic agent the liver cannot remove from the blood ends up in the kidneys and skin. Nephrologists and other health care providers need to be aware of certain medications and diagnostic test preparations that, in some patients, can cause damage to the kidneys, according to a special clinical update being presented at the American Society of Nephrology's 40th Annual Meeting and Scientific Exposition in San Francisco.

The four presentations in this special Clinical Nephrology Conference (CNC) draw attention to several recently recognized 'iatrogenic' (caused by medical treatments or tests) kidney disorders. Some of the problems are related to widely used products, including bisphosphonate drugs used to treat osteoporosis and 'bowel prep' solution used to prepare for colonoscopy.

Dr. Daniel W. Coyne of Washington University School of Medicine, St. Louis, Mo. discusses the risk of kidney disorders associated with the use of bisphosphonates. Increasing evidence suggests that in some circumstances, these widely used osteoporosis drugs can cause certain types of kidney damage. The risks are higher with 'nitrogen-containing' types of bisphosphonate drugs and may depend on the individual patient and the total dose over time. Fortunately, the kidney damage is usually reversible after bisphosphonate treatment has stopped.

Despite these risks, bisphosphonates are still used for the purpose of treating the high rate of osteoporosis in patients with kidney disease. Recent studies have even suggested that bisphosphonates can slow the buildup of calcium deposits in the blood vessels of patients on dialysis.

When the basic renal and hepatic excretory systems fail, the skin, being an alternate route for the excretion of undesirable substances, automatically bears the brunt of the systemic toxicity.

Once overburdened with these internal, highly acidic toxins, the skin becomes vulnerable to the natural elements, including sunlight. Skin cancer and cataracts only occur if the liver is congested.

It is much easier to treat the cause of a physical problem than to suppress its symptoms. If you are taking any of the above drugs and wish to treat the cause rather than the effect of an illness, consult with your doctor about how to phase them out gradually, cleanse your elimination organs, and at the same time begin exposing your body to the sun, starting with 1 or 2 minutes and building up a few more minutes each day. Make certain, though, that your skin doesn't get burned. If you wear sunglasses, expose your eyes to natural light for as long as it is comfortable. Try to restrict your use to only when the glare is reflected off snow or the road. Gradually you will wean yourself from sunglasses and will no longer require them. To avoid dehydration of the skin, drink fresh water before and after exposure to the sun.

CHAPTER 10:
Sunlight Prevents Cancer, MS, Heart Disease, Arthritis, Diabetes...

According to a study published in the prominent *Cancer* journal *(March 2002; 94:1867-75)*, insufficient exposure to ultraviolet radiation may be an important risk factor for cancer in Western Europe and North America.

The findings, covering mortality rates from cancer in North America, directly contradict official advice about sunlight. The research showed that deaths from a range of cancers of the reproductive and digestive systems were approximately twice as high in New England as in the Southwest, despite a diet that varied little between the two regions. An examination of 506 regions found a close inverse correlation between cancer mortality and levels of UVB light.

The likeliest mechanism proposed by scientists for a protective effect from sunlight is vitamin D, which is synthesized by the body when exposed to ultraviolet B rays. According to the study's author, Dr William Grant, the northern parts of the United States may be dark enough during the winter months such that vitamin D synthesis shuts down completely. While the study focused mainly on white Americans, it also found that the same geographical trend affects black or darker skinned Americans, whose overall cancer rates are significantly higher. As explained earlier, darker skinned people require more sunlight to synthesize vitamin D. The study showed at least 13 malignancies affected by lack of sunlight, mostly reproductive and digestive cancers. The strongest inverse correlation is with breast, colon, and ovarian cancer, followed by tumors of the bladder, uterus, esophagus, rectum, and stomach.

What is vitamin D?

Vitamin D, calciferol, is a fat-soluble vitamin. It can be obtained from certain foodstuffs, but is chiefly synthesized in the body after exposure to ultraviolet rays from the sun.

Vitamin D exists in different forms. Vitamin D obtained from sun exposure, food, and supplements, is biologically inert and must undergo two hydroxylation reactions to be activated in the body. Calcitriol (1,25-Dihydroxycholecalciferol) is the active form of vitamin D found in the body.

The major biologic function of vitamin D is to maintain normal blood levels of calcium and phosphorus. Vitamin D aids in the absorption of calcium and promotes bone mineralization in concert with a number of other vitamins, minerals, and hormones.

Vitamin D can be acquired through exposure to sunlight or through dietary intake. Sunlight is the most important source for the synthesis of vitamin D. Ultraviolet (UV) rays from sunlight trigger vitamin D synthesis in the skin. Fortified foods are the major dietary sources of vitamin D.

Most people are aware of the significance of vitamin D in the maintenance of healthy bones. What people fail to realize is that the role of vitamin D is not limited to the prevention of bone diseases/disorders alone. Vitamin D can also prevent several other diseases - autoimmune diseases like Rheumatoid Arthritis (RA), Multiple Sclerosis (MS) Diabetes Mellitus (DM), cancers, heart disease etc.

Vitamin D and MS:

There are few effective treatments for the neurologic problem called Multiple Sclerosis. Sufferers tend to get progressively worse and often end up in wheelchairs, unable to even perform the simplest tasks by themselves. But a new study is showing that effective treatment is right outside the door - in the form of the inexpensive and even FREE - Vitamin D.

Multiple Sclerosis is a devastating disease with few treatment options except hope. It often strikes at a young age and leaves the afflicted people unable to care for themselves when they should be in the prime of their lives. It gets its name from the 'sclerosed' appearance that the fatty outer layer of the spinal cord, the myelin sheath, has when viewed on medical scans. These patches slow down - and even stop - electrical transmissions from the brain to the rest of the body and vice versa. Over time, strength and movement slow down and are lost entirely.

Treatments for multiple sclerosis haven't worked very well, but drug manufacturers and researchers are always attempting to develop treatments to, if not cure the disease, at least give sufferers relief from their symptoms. Some drug treatments that have seemed to show promise are, as usual, being found to have serious consequences like brain infections from the drug Rituximab and an increase in cancer from a class of drugs called beta interferons!

Interferons have been used widely for the treatment of MS, a neurological disease, for almost a decade, and are available, along with glatiramer acetateon for this use, free of charge from many national health services. However, the long-term effectiveness of both drugs has not been confirmed and any beneficial effects might be outweighed by their side effects and high costs.

In an analysis of trials conducted so far on the use of interferon in patients with the relapsing-remitting form of MS, interferon had a 'modest' protective effect during the first year of treatment. However, results could not be determined for the second year due to trial weaknesses, including high dropout rates and little to no follow-up of patients, and differences in reporting of methods.

Side effects were greater among patients taking interferon than those taking a placebo. Flu-like symptoms were common and the occurrence of leucopenia, lymphocytopenia, thrombocytopenia, and raised liver enzymes in blood was higher than controls.

Scientists conclude that while interferon may have a modest effect during the first year of treatment, its effectiveness beyond one year is not known. Despite this, patients are commonly treated with interferon for long time periods. Scientists say that the drug's effectiveness should be assessed.

But it seems that MS sufferers may not have to make that choice any more. A new study shows that those taking VERY high doses of Vitamin D, about 14,000 IUs per day on average, prevented the frequent relapses that occur with the disease. These high doses of Vitamin D significantly helped the patients in the study to maintain their current level of functioning with virtually no adverse effects. It is somewhat baffling that the researchers warned other MS sufferers not to take more than 4000 IUs of Vitamin D per day until the treatment was proven to be safe.

This is baffling for two reasons: one because the much lower dosages of 4,000 IUs that were used in the study showed absolutely no benefit; and two because study after study has already shown that high dose Vitamin D is safe. In fact the University of Toronto, the research facility for this study, had stated previously in a different study that there is "no evidence of adverse effects from taking 10,000 IU of Vitamin D a day".

But even if you are skeptical about taking high doses of Vitamin D in pill form, where there is the chance of taking too much, you can get a high dose Vitamin D for free just by exposing your skin to sunlight. If you are light-skinned and expose the majority of your body to direct sunlight for the amount of time that it takes you to get the slightest bit pink, you will make up to 20,000 IUs of Vitamin D. Interestingly, even though the body makes such a large amount of Vitamin D all at once, there has never been a recorded overdose of Vitamin D from too much sun.

While this may be the first study to show the effectiveness of Vitamin D to prevent relapses in MS, there is already precedent for the use of Vitamin D in the disease. Several studies have shown that higher levels of Vitamin D are effective at preventing Multiple Sclerosis in the first place. Another study showed that the number of sclerosed areas on the spinal cord could be reduced by as much as HALF using the same high dose Vitamin D used in this study!! In fact, Vitamin D researchers such as Oliver Gilley, who did extensive studies on Scotland's high rate of Multiple Sclerosis, has been urging higher levels of Vitamin D for years in order to ward off this preventable disease.

So, while drug researchers continue looking for the latest and greatest drug treatments, Great Britain urges its Prime Minister to devote millions of pounds for stem cell research and the Multiple Sclerosis Society of Canada creates new training centers designed to "conduct MS research through training of the next generation of MS researchers"; the 'next generation' for the prevention and treatment of this 'incurable' disease is sitting right in front of us - right here, right now. While you may have to weigh the risks and benefits of getting your Vitamin D through the sun, this safe and effective treatment for Multiple Sclerosis is completely free of charge and no insurance is required.

According to a study, women who take vitamin D supplements through multivitamins are 40 percent less likely to develop multiple sclerosis (MS) than women who do not take supplements. The study, which involved 187,563 women, is the first examination to question if MS is caused by lack of sunlight, which prevents the body from making its own vitamin D.

Researchers examined data collected from two large studies involving the women, one was a 20-year-old study and the other was a 10-year-old study. The participants' diets and use of multivitamin supplements were measured in the beginning of the study and then again every four years. Out of the 187,563 women participating in the study, 173 developed MS during the course of it.

Researchers divided the large group of women into groups based on vitamin D use. The study found that the risk of developing MS was lower both for those with high intakes of vitamin D supplements (400 IU or more per day) and for those with high intakes from the supplements and food. However, the study also suggested that the participants whose intake of vitamin D was only from food did not have any lesser risk of developing MS.

Evidence continues to mount showing that a little vitamin D can do a lot more than build strong bones. We have known for some time that vitamin D can affect function of the immune system, which could explain why it seems beneficial in this autoimmune condition.

Although most MS patients have a normal life span, the disease, which causes the immune system to attack the body's own cells as 'foreign', causes vision changes and muscle weakness in its victims. MS may progress steadily, or acute attacks may be followed by a temporary remission of symptoms.

We need adequate amounts of vitamin D to keep cell growth and activity in check. When the body is deficient in this crucial nutrient - best known for coming from sunlight - cells can go haywire, become overly active or multiply too quickly. These results are not too surprising though as it has been well-known that if you live at higher latitudes, where there is less sun exposure, you are at a higher risk of developing MS. Conversely, if you live in a sunny climate where vitamin D can easily be absorbed year-round from sunlight for your first 10 years, it imprints on you a decreased MS risk that can last a lifetime.

In a recently published exploratory study, mortality from multiple sclerosis (MS) was found to be reduced by exposure to sunlight. Depending on the degree of sunlight exposure, the risk of death from MS was reduced by up to 76%. No theory on the precise mechanism of action in this reduction was proposed by the authors. (Occup Environ Med 2000;57:418-421)

Children and adolescents who had high sun exposure had a decreased risk of multiple sclerosis (MS) later in life. Researchers concluded that insufficient exposure to ultraviolet radiation or vitamin D might therefore increase the risk of MS. Other studies have had similar results, indicating that ultraviolet radiation may be beneficial against multiple sclerosis.

Sun exposure during childhood and early adolescence seemed to be most effective against MS, researchers found. Further, higher sun exposure during winter months, when minimum ultraviolet radiation and vitamin D exposures occur, was particularly important in reducing the risk of MS. (British Medical Journal August 9, 2003;327:316)

Vitamin D and heart disease:

Researchers in Belgium appear to be the first to have shown that simple, natural and cheap vitamin D (cholecalciferol) lowers C - Reactive Protein (CRP), a measure of inflammation in the body, in critically ill patients.

Even small amounts of vitamin D, about 500 IU, lowered inflammation by more than 25 % in a small group of critically ill patients. Another marker of inflammation (IL-6) was reduced even more. The researchers also found that critically ill patients were profoundly deficient in vitamin D.

In another study, researchers found that vitamin D deficiency is associated with increased inflammation in otherwise healthy people. Increased inflammation in the body can increase the risk of chronic inflammatory conditions, including coronary heart disease (CHD) and diabetes. Further, the researchers found that inflammation was lowered by simple vitamin D.

As vitamin D deficiency is associated with numerous illnesses with inflammatory components, such as hypertension, heart disease, diabetes, autoimmune illness and heart disease, the findings were important. The authors concluded: "This finding provides a possible mechanism for tissue damage in chronic inflammatory conditions, including CHD and diabetes."

Inflammation in the body may be as important as cholesterol in determining the risk of heart disease. Unlike cholesterol alone, cholesterol and inflammation together predict a substantial number of cases of heart disease.

Various studies show that vitamin D deficiency is widespread among the critically ill and suggest that that this may contribute to the inflammatory basis of various illnesses.

For example, researchers studied patients with congestive heart failure and found elevated levels of TNF, another marker of inflammation. They also found critically low levels of calcidiol [25(OH)D], the only reliable marker of vitamin D, and even found low levels of calcitriol, the active form of vitamin D that is usually low only in those who are severely vitamin D deficient.

They concluded that vitamin D deficiency might contribute to the development of congestive heart failure (CHF).

It is important to note that vitamin D's anti-inflammatory actions in humans have long been suspected. For example, several studies using compounds similar to vitamin D have been shown to significantly reduce inflammation and improve the patients' condition when given to patients suffering from rheumatoid arthritis.

Studies show that a lack of vitamin D may even contribute to congestive heart failure, as researchers found that patients with chronic heart failure have lower levels of the vitamin in the blood.

Congestive heart failure occurs when the heart fails to pump blood around the body efficiently and organs are not able to get enough nutrients and oxygen.

Previous animal research has indicated a link between vitamin D and heart failure, which spurred researchers to conduct the study on humans.

54 patients with chronic heart failure (CHF) were compared with 34 healthy people, and it was found that CHF patients had vitamin D levels that were up to 50 % lower than healthy patients. It was noted that the more severe the vitamin D deficiency, the worse the heart failure symptoms.

According to researchers, vitamin D may play a role in regulating calcium concentration in cells of the heart muscle. If calcium concentration is not controlled, muscle cells cannot expand and contract properly, which means that blood will not be pumped efficiently around the body.

Humans make vitamin D, but the majority is synthesized from sun exposure. Lack of sun exposure, which is an increasing problem as people spend long hours in offices or in front of television sets, can result in vitamin D deficiency.

The value of Vitamin D in having a healthy heart is remarkable. It is useful in a number of ways including :-

• Blood pressure regulation:- While there is no direct evidence that vitamin D supplementation will lower blood pressure, people with high blood pressure generally have low blood levels of vitamin D.

• Heart attack, stroke, heart failure reduction:- A recent study in Circulation reported that events such as heart attacks, strokes, and heart failure were anywhere from 53% to 80% higher in people with low levels of vitamin D in their blood. That risk increased even more in people with high blood pressure. Low blood levels of vitamin D may increase the risk of heart disease and stroke, especially for people with high blood pressure, according to researchers with the Framingham Heart Study. The scientists followed 1,739 men and women for more than 5 years and reported that participants with low blood levels of vitamin D were 62% more likely to develop cardiovascular disease than those with higher levels. For those with low vitamin D levels and high blood pressure, cardiovascular risk doubled.

• Helps reduce inflammation:- Researchers speculate that more vitamin D could lead to less inflammation in the arteries. Until recently, most researchers believed that heart disease was essentially a 'plumbing' problem caused by an accumulation of hardened fat and cholesterol in the coronary arteries, known as plaque. However, an increasing body of evidence now shows that this accumulation of plaque is actually the result of chronic, low-grade inflammation in the coronary arteries. Researchers also believe that in the battle against heart disease, damping down this inflammation is nearly as important as lowering cholesterol.

Vitamin D and DM:

In Norway, cod liver oil has been an important dietary source of vitamin D because it contains the biological properties that were critical for the prevention of type 1 diabetes. *[Note: Although cod liver oil is an excellent source of vitamin D, I personally don't endorse it because it has shown to have toxic effects on the liver.]*

A study was conducted to find out whether the intake of dietary cod liver oil or other sources of vitamin D such as supplements taken by either mothers during pregnancy or by children during the first year of their life was linked to lowering the risk of type 1 diabetes among children.

The nationwide case-control study was done in Norway and consisted of 545 children diagnosed with type 1 diabetes and 1,668 control participants. Families were sent a questionnaire in the mail and were required to answer questions pertaining to the number of times they used cod liver oil or other vitamin D supplements.

Results from the study showed that taking cod liver oil during the first year of life greatly lowered the risk of type 1 diabetes. The consumption of other vitamin D supplements during the first year of life and pregnancy were not connected with type 1 diabetes.

The study concluded that the anti-inflammatory effects of long-chain omega-3 fatty acids found in cod liver oil might have the capability of reducing the risk of type 1 diabetes. (American Journal Clinical Nutrition May 2004;79:820-5)

Exposure to the sun is a far more preferable way to receive your vitamin D than taking it from a pill or liquid. Using a UV lamp or vitamin D lamp or safe tanning bed is the second best option. If you don't have any other choice, then by all means use a vitamin D supplement, but it is extremely important to have your vitamin D levels checked to avoid toxicity.

Vitamin D and musculoskeletal disease:

It is estimated that over 25 million adults in the United States have, or are at risk of developing osteoporosis. Osteoporosis is a disease characterized by fragile bones. It results in increased risk of bone fractures.

Rickets and osteomalacia were recognized as being caused by vitamin D deficiency 75 years ago; their prevention and cure with fish liver oil constituted one of the early triumphs of nutritional science. The requirement for vitamin D has been pegged to these disorders ever since.

Having normal storage levels of vitamin D in your body helps keep your bones strong and may help prevent osteoporosis in elderly, non-ambulatory individuals, in post-menopausal women, and in individuals on chronic steroid therapy.

Researchers know that normal bone is constantly being remodeled (broken down and rebuilt). During menopause, when typically previously unnoticed physical imbalance become apparent, the balance between these two processes is upset, resulting in more bone being broken down (resorbed) than rebuilt.

Vitamin D deficiency has been associated with greater incidence of hip fractures. A higher vitamin D concentration in the blood has been associated with less bone loss in older women. Since bone loss increases the risk of fractures, increased vitamin D presence in the body may help prevent fractures resulting from osteoporosis.

The beneficial effect of vitamin D is well accepted, but the mere absence of clinical rickets can hardly be considered an adequate definition either of health or of vitamin D sufficiency.

The fact that it takes 30 or more years to manifest itself, makes it no less a deficiency condition than a disorder that develops in 30 days. It is easy to understand how long-period deficiency diseases could never have been recognized in the early days of nutritional science, but with modern methods and a better grasp of the relevant physiology, failing to recognize a slowly developing condition as a true deficiency state, can no longer be justified.

Vitamin D nutrition probably affects major aspects of human health, as listed below, other than its classical role in mineral metabolism. The rest of the article addresses some of the newly-recognized uses of vitamin D.

Rickets appears to be on the rise, particularly in African-American children, according to a new report. Rickets is a disorder most commonly caused by vitamin D deficiency that results in soft, malformed bones, and muscle weakness.

Researchers reviewed medical records of 30 babies diagnosed with nutritional rickets between 1990 and 1999 at two medical centers in North Carolina.

All of the children were African-American, aged 5 months to 25 months, and all were breast-fed but did not receive vitamin D supplements.

Over half of the patients were seen in 1998 and the first half of 1999, giving the researchers the impression that the incidence has risen sharply. At the time of diagnosis, most of the infants were growth retarded in both height and weight with nearly one-third being severely growth retarded. Many of the infants also had bow legs and bone fractures, common problems with untreated vitamin D deficiency.

Vitamin D comes from two sources: food and sunlight. Some of the richest food sources of vitamin D are liver, egg yolks, and fish. The natural vitamin D in butter was found 100 times as effective as the common commercial form of D (viosterol), according to early research (Supplee, G. C., Ansbacher, S., Bender, R. C., and Flanigan, G. E., "The Influence of Milk Constituents on the Effectiveness of Vitamin D," Journal of Biological Chemistry, 141:95?107, May, 1936). In addition, butter, prescribed by physicians as a remedy for tuberculosis, psoriasis, xerophthalmia, dental caries, and in preventing rickets, has been promptly effective.

Besides butter, especially medicinal mushrooms, such as Reishi, Krestin, Cordyceps, Maitake, Ganoderma Lucidum,

Shiitake and all other natural mushrooms contain much vitamin D. If exposed to the sun for five minutes, their vitamin D content becomes multiplied, not much different to when we expose our skin to the sun.

Researchers suggest that there are several possible causes for the rise of infant rickets:

- The increasing proportion of women who breastfeed their babies:- Although experts encourage breastfeeding, the vitamin D content of breast milk depends on the mother having adequate levels of the vitamin. (Typically, breast milk tends to have very low levels of vitamin D, usually not enough to meet the needs of an exclusively breastfed baby.)
- Pediatricians may not be adequately prescribing vitamin supplements for infants, especially to those who are breastfed.
- Dark-skinned people are more prone to vitamin D deficiencies because dark skin requires more sunlight to manufacture vitamin D, but the researchers stress that rickets is completely preventable.

Breastfeeding is definitely the ideal source of nutrition for babies and children, but supplementation of dark-skinned, breast-fed infants and children with 400 IU of vitamin D per day, starting at least by 2 months of age is necessary.

Many breastfeeding advocates are justifiably defensive of any perceived defamation of breastfeeding, and therefore disagree with the assertion that vitamin D supplementation is required in a breastfed baby. This objection may actually derive from the very appropriate advocacy for human milk as a 'perfect food'. It IS the perfect food.

Unfortunately for some, the very need for supplementation may be interpreted as a nutritional inadequacy in breast milk. As emphasized above, however, calciferol (vitamin D) is in no sense to be looked at as a nutrient, but rather the precursor of a steroid hormone that is not naturally present in any infant food. Classifying the anti-rachitic substance in cod liver oil as a vitamin was an unfortunate historical error that has become too ingrained to correct.

If one views calciferol in this light, then it is not necessary to consider human milk 'deficient'. Instead, the provision of supplemental calciferol can be looked on as ensuring an adequate substrate for a hormone whose normal production has been adversely affected by the realities of modern living conditions. Human milk is, indeed, the 'perfect food' for infants. Unfortunately, neither it nor any non-supplemented food or formula can prevent climate, latitude, smog, economic factors, or religious practices from coming between infants and sunshine. (Journal of Pediatrics August 2000; 137: 153-157.)

Vitamin D is NOT a vitamin but a steroid hormone precursor that is NOT naturally present in food. This explains why the most perfect food on the planet for humans, human breast milk, is 'deficient' in vitamin D.

Vitamin D is one of the only supplements that a breastfed baby will need, but this is only if the baby is not exposed to sunshine. The darker the skin of the baby, the more sun exposure will be required for the baby to generate enough vitamin D. Even if the child does not develop rickets, less than optimal bone development and other problems will occur without adequate vitamin D. Typically, parents are so concerned about calcium for proper bone growth and health, but in most cases the vitamin D is far more important.

Researchers have linked vitamin D concentrations greater than 40 nmol/L with improved lower extremity function in ambulatory patients aged 60 and older, regardless of calcium intake, activity level, sex, age, race or ethnicity.

Many young adults are not getting enough vitamin D, particularly during the winter months. Young adults aged 18 to 29 years have an equal to greater risk of vitamin D insufficiency than do older adults, especially during the winter. This is one of the first studies in the United States revealing a relatively high prevalence of vitamin D insufficiency in young adults. Vitamin D, which helps the body to absorb calcium, is made by the body when the skin is exposed to sunlight. Vitamin D deficiency puts people at risk for the bone-thinning disease osteoporosis as well as chronic bone and muscle pains, and may also increase the risk of certain cancers.

To investigate vitamin D insufficiency, the researchers screened 165 men and women during March and April, at the end of winter, and 142 individuals during September and October, at the end of summer. Young adults had a 30% increase in their vitamin D levels from the end of winter to the end of summer. Nearly two-thirds of the end-of-summer group and 58% of the end-of-winter group reported drinking almost two glasses of milk per day, but this was not associated with higher vitamin D levels. On the other hand, the 4 out of 10 study participants who reported taking daily multivitamin supplements during the summer and winter months had vitamin D levels 30% higher than those who did not take the supplements. (The American Journal of Medicine June 2002;112:659-662)

The numbers for vitamin D deficiency are actually far worse than this study has reported because researchers are using dated optimum levels of vitamin D. They are using reference ranges from the sun-deprived US populations, while they should be using reference ranges established from people who live in sub-tropical environments with regular sun exposure.

The fact that the vitamin D from milk did not help to improve low vitamin D level should not be surprising because the vitamin D in milk is synthetic vitamin D2 (ergocalciferol) which is not effective at replacing vitamin D as the natural vitamin D3 (cholecalciferol) that is received from the sun, natural butter or medicinal mushrooms. D2 is a form not found naturally in humans, and therefore is of no benefit. It is a huge money maker, though, and a scam.

CHAPTER 11:
The Sun Cuts Cancer Risk by Half or More!

In the 1940s, Frank Apperly demonstrated a link between latitude and deaths from cancer. He suggested that sunlight provided people with a relative cancer immunity. This is now a proven fact.

According to two recent studies conducted at the University of San Diego, increasing blood levels of vitamin D through sunlight may decrease a person's risk of developing breast cancer by 50 % and of developing colorectal cancer by more than 65 %.

To increase the precision and accuracy of the study, researchers used meta-analysis to pool data from multiple previous studies. They divided subjects into groups based on their blood levels of vitamin D and compared the incidence of cancer between groups. The collected data showed that individuals in the group with the lowest blood levels of vitamin D had the highest rates of breast cancer, and the breast cancer rates dropped as the blood levels increased. The most astounding finding in this study is that the blood level associated with a 50 % lower risk of breast cancer could be reached by spending as little as 25 minutes in the sun for darker skinned people, and no more than 10 to 15 minutes for lighter skinned individuals. This practically makes the sun an instant healer, far more effective than even the most aggressively hyped cancer drugs, such as Herceptin. The second study showed that the same amount of sunlight corresponded with a two-thirds lower risk of contracting colorectal cancer. For any doctor or friend who asks for proof for the 'outrageous' claim that sunlight can prevent or cure cancer, you may want to refer him or her to the *Journal of Steroid Biochemistry and Molecular Biology* (doi: 10.1016/j.jsbmb.2006.12.007; 'Vitamin D and prevention of breast cancer: Pooled analysis') and to the *American Journal of Preventive Medicine* (Volume 32, Number 3, Pages 210-

216 'Optimal vitamin status for colorectal cancer prevention - A quantitative meta-analysis').

Results of one small study suggested that body stores of vitamin D may be associated with survival chances in women with advanced breast cancer. "13 women with normal or high levels of active vitamin D survived the 6-month test period but, sadly, in those with low levels, 5 out of 13 died within 6 months," said Professor Barbara Mawer of the Manchester Royal Infirmary in central England.

Exciting new research conducted at the Creighton University School of Medicine in Nebraska has revealed that supplementing with vitamin D and calcium can reduce your risk of cancer by an astonishing 77 %. This includes breast cancer, colon cancer, skin cancer and other forms of cancer. This research provides strong new evidence that vitamin D is the single most effective medicine against cancer, far outpacing the benefits of any cancer drug known to modern science.

The study involved 1,179 healthy women from rural Nebraska. One group of women was given calcium (around 1500 mg daily) and vitamin D (1100 IU daily) while another group was given placebo. Over four year, the group receiving the calcium and vitamin D supplements showed a 60 % decrease in cancers. Considering just the last 3 years of the study reveals an impressive 77 % reduction in cancer due to supplementation.

This research on vitamin D is such good news that the American Cancer Society, of course, had to say something against it. An ACS spokesperson, Marji McCullough, strategic director of nutritional epidemiology for the American Cancer Society, flatly stated that nobody should take supplements to prevent cancer.

If it seems surprising to you that the American Cancer Society - which claims to be against cancer - would dissuade people from taking supplements that slash their cancer risk by 77 %, then you don't know much about the ACS. The ACS is an organization that actually prevents prevention and openly supports the continuation of cancer as a way to boost its power and profits. The ACS is the wealthiest non-profit organization in America and has very close ties to pharmaceutical companies, mammography equipment companies and other corporations that profit from cancer.

According to another study, women with breast cancer are twice as likely to have a fault in the gene required to make use of vitamin D. Experts already believe vitamin D protects against breast cancer and in some forms may even be used to shrink existing tumors.

Now research in London suggests that women with genetic variations (polymorphisms) of the vitamin D receptor gene may be less able to benefit from this protective effect.

Researchers said the study added to the increasing evidence for a role of vitamin D receptor gene polymorphisms in the cancer disease process.

While vitamin D and its analogues are being developed as preventative and/or treatment agents in breast cancer, the assessment of vitamin D receptor polymorphisms may be vital in the identification of at-risk groups and strategies for targeting and intervention.

She stressed that a screening test was not worthwhile in the present state of knowledge and that women should not suddenly start taking lots of vitamin D tablets.

There has been a great deal of research into vitamin D and its effects on cancer, and some potential new cancer treatments are based on vitamin D. This study is very important because it may help us identify more women who are at risk from breast cancer and gives us more clues on how to treat them.

An article in the British medical journal *Lancet* offers evidence that lack of vitamin D causes prostate cancer. Most men meet their needs for vitamin D through exposure to sunlight because they do not get enough from their diet. Men who live in colder climates have a higher incidence of prostate cancer because they get less sunlight. Studies from the Harvard School of Public Health show that men who drink more than four glasses of milk a day, have low blood levels of vitamin D and have an increased risk for prostate cancer. Calcium uses up vitamin D and not enough vitamin D is added to milk to cover the extra calcium used. Besides, synthetic vitamin D is quite difficult to absorb.

This study shows that prostate cancer is associated with not exposing skin to sunlight and not going on holidays to beach resorts. Susceptibility to prostate cancer was not found to be associated with vasectomy, benign prostatic enlargement or eating any particular food.

New research suggests that vitamin D may protect against colon cancer also by helping to get rid of a toxic acid that promotes the disease.

The discovery could point the way to the development of therapies that provide the cancer protection of vitamin D without the side effects caused by consuming too much of the vitamin.

Now we believe that we have discovered the potential mechanism of how vitamin D can be protective of colon cancer. If it is not the only mechanism, it is at least one of them.

Vitamin D is known to protect against colon cancer, but exactly how has been uncertain. The high-fat 'Western' diet has been linked to an increased risk of the disease, although this connection is controversial.

The new research provides a possible explanation for the protection of vitamin D as well as the increased risk of a high-fat diet. Researchers found that vitamin D and a type of bile acid called lithocholic acid (LCA) both activate the vitamin D receptor in cells.

When a person eats fatty foods, the liver empties bile acids into the intestine, making it possible for the body to absorb fatty substances. After doing their job in the intestine, most bile acids are taken back into the liver.

But LCA does something unusual. It is not re-circulated into the liver. Instead, an enzyme called CYP3A degrades LCA in the intestine. If LCA is not detoxified by the enzyme, it passes into the colon where it can promote cancer. LCA is very toxic.

Since vitamin D has been shown to prevent colon cancer in animals, the researchers decided to see whether its receptor had any effect on the detoxification of LCA.

In fact, the vitamin D receptor seems to act as a sensor for high levels of LCA. The vitamin D receptor binds to LCA, triggering an increase in the expression of the gene for CYP3A, the acid-neutralizing enzyme. This seems to be the body's way of protecting itself from colon cancer.

If a person does not get enough vitamin D, this balance may be interrupted, increasing the risk of colon cancer.

The research also provides a possible explanation of how high-fat diets may increase the risk of colon cancer. Since LCA is released from the liver when a person eats fatty food, a high-fat diet that keeps LCA levels high may 'overwhelm the system'. The body may stop producing enough CYP3A to keep LCA under control.

Unlike drugs, surgery or radiation, sunlight costs nothing, has no harmful side-effects, and can prevent numerous other diseases at the same time. Not dissimilar to the study on cancers, researchers found a strong correlation between geography and multiple sclerosis (MS). As it turns out, the incidence of MS decreases the closer to the equator (where the most UV sunlight is) one resides.

Children who develop multiple sclerosis have substantially lower levels of vitamin D than children who do not develop the disease, according to a series of studies presented at an international conference on multiple sclerosis in Montreal.

Multiple sclerosis is a degenerative disease of the nervous system in which the myelin sheath that insulates nerve cells breaks down, leading to problems in the transmission of nervous signals. Symptoms can range from tingling and numbness to tremors, paralysis or blindness. An estimated 2.5 million people around the world suffer from the disease, which is rarely diagnosed before the age of 15.

In one study, researchers from the University of Toronto tested the vitamin D blood levels of 125 children who had exhibited symptoms indicating some form of damage to the myelin sheath.

"Three-quarters of our subjects were below the optimal levels for vitamin D," said lead researcher Heather Hanwell.

After a year, the researchers compared the data from the 20 children who had since been diagnosed with multiple sclerosis with those who had not exhibited any further demyelinating symptoms. They found that the average vitamin D levels of children who had been diagnosed with multiple sclerosis were substantially lower than those of the other children. Among the diagnosed children, 68 % of children were actually deficient in the vitamin.

A similar study was conducted by researchers from Toronto's Hospital for Sick Children.

"17 of 19 children who had been diagnosed with MS had vitamin D levels below the target level," said researcher Brenda Banwell.

Researchers have suspected a connection between vitamin D and multiple sclerosis for many years, ever since discovering that the disease is more common at more northern latitudes. Because the body synthesizes vitamin D upon exposure to sunlight, deficiency is much more common in places where the sun is weaker, especially during the winter.

"There is a very consistent pattern of latitude and multiple sclerosis," said epidemiologist and multiple sclerosis researcher Cedric Garland of the University of California-San Diego.

Hanwell directly linked Canada's northern latitude to its high rates of multiple sclerosis. "In Canada for 6 months of the year, the sun is not intense enough for us to manufacture vitamin D in our skin," she said.

Canada has one of the highest multiple sclerosis rates in the world. One of the few countries with a higher rate is Scotland, which has regions reached by only a quarter of all available sunlight. Recent research has confirmed a strong connection in Scotland between vitamin D deficiency and poor health status.

"People have been looking for things in the environment that might account for why Canada has such a high MS risk, and this is one of those factors," said Banwell.

It remains unclear exactly how vitamin D might influence multiple sclerosis risk, but researchers believe it may have to do with the immune system. New research continues to illuminate the role that vitamin D plays in the immune system, providing protection against cancer, tuberculosis and autoimmune diseases.

Many health researchers believe that multiple sclerosis is an autoimmune disease.

"Vitamin D acts as an immune modulator," said Banwell. "On our immune cells, there are, what are known as receptors, a docking mechanism, for vitamin D. In MS, there are many lines of evidence that immune cells are not regulated properly."

The American National Institute of Health (NIH) has linked deficiencies of the sun-made vitamin D to rising rates of many diseases, including osteoporosis, rheumatoid arthritis, heart disease, and diabetes, just to name a few.

There are several diseases and conditions caused by vitamin D deficiency.

- Osteoporosis is commonly caused by a lack of vitamin D, which greatly impairs calcium absorption. Sufficient vitamin D prevents prostate cancer, breast cancer, ovarian cancer, depression, colon cancer and schizophrenia.
- 'Rickets' is the name of the bone-wasting disease caused by vitamin D deficiency.
- Vitamin D deficiency may exacerbate type 2 Diabetes and impair insulin production in the pancreas.

105

- Obesity impairs vitamin D utilization in the body, meaning obese people need twice as much vitamin D.
- Vitamin D is used around the world to treat Psoriasis.
- Vitamin D deficiency is also linked with schizophrenia.
- Seasonal Affective Disorder is caused by a melatonin imbalance initiated by lack of exposure to sunlight.
- Chronic vitamin D deficiency is often misdiagnosed as fibromyalgia because its symptoms are so similar: muscle weakness, aches and pains.
- Your risk of developing serious diseases like diabetes and cancer is reduced by 50-80% through simple, sensible exposure to natural sunlight 2-3 times each week.
- Infants who receive vitamin D supplementation (2000 units daily) have an 80% reduced risk of developing type 1 diabetes over the next 20 years.

Today, up to 60% of all hospital patients and up to 80% of all nursing home patients are vitamin D deficient. What is worse is that 76% of pregnant mothers are severely vitamin D deficient. To get the disease-curbing benefits of sunlight, you need to get outside at least three times a week, for a minimum of 15-20 minutes each time. Pharmaceutical companies have also recognized the importance of vitamin D in the cure of cancer and other illnesses and now produce expensive drugs that contain synthetic Vitamin D.

However, synthetic vitamin D has little or no effect when compared with vitamin D produced by sunlight. In addition, vitamin D added to foods such as milk, can cause serious side effects that include death. (*See details in 'Vitamin Euphoria', Chapter 14 of Timeless Secrets of Health and Rejuvenation*)

CHAPTER 12:
The Amazing Sunlight/Exercise Combination

Exercise and sunlight as two separate entities are both essential for good health.

What significance does exercise have in healthy living?

Exercising daily is important to maintain physical, emotional, mental, social, and spiritual health.

Exercise alone is good, no doubt, but let us talk about why exercising out in the sun is better. Why do I think it is important to encourage exercise outdoors in the sun? The environment indoors is far from the healthiest to exercise in or for that matter to perform most activities in. So long as the air outside is fresh and pollution-free, the outdoor environment is ideal for exercise. Apart from the energizing and nourishing aspect of sunshine on our fiber, it also emotionally charges us and serves to invigorate the mind. It is no surprise then that in late winter a lot of people go into depressed states and suffer from what is often referred to as cabin fever or more appropriately seasonal affective disorder[5] (SAD). During those long winter days when isolated indoors, the body fails to receive the much required (and often on a subconscious level - craved) sunshine and predisposes one to SAD. The only cure, relief and mode of prevention can be found in sunlight (limited though it may be). The amount of sunshine each person needs depends on each person's body and constitution. Accordingly, the length of time required must differ. The essential thing is to get as much of the nourishing sun during these periods as possible.

---

[5]Seasonal Affective Disorder (SAD), also known as winter depression or winter blues, is a mood disorder in which people who have normal mental health throughout most of the year experience depressive symptoms in the winter or, less frequently, in the summer, spring or autumn, repeatedly, year after year. In the Diagnostic and Statistical Manual of Mental Disorders (DSM-IV), SAD is not a unique mood disorder, but is "a specifier of major depression".

Coming back to the significance of exercise, as we all know, exercise involves motion and motion is natural, all animals move, and so must we. Staying glued to a place for long periods is unhealthy. You need to get out and move about. Exercise is what gives your muscles tone and strength and keeps your weight in check, curbs your anxiety and works as a remarkable antidepressant.

Exercise stimulates cognitive function. Exercise can radically prevent or delay the deterioration of mental faculties as age progresses especially in the late years. It boosts circulation all over the body and the brain tissue is not exempted from the blood flood. Exercise is an absolute energizing experience. Opiate-like hormones called endorphins and encephalins, known to be released during exercise contribute to the 'exercise high', that feel-good factor associated with exercise when done regularly. The rhythmic breathing and collective consciousness during exercise can also be a spiritually uplifting experience. We now realize that a healthy diet, good hygiene and clean environment alone cannot and do not ensure good health; exercise is just as vital.

The benefits of sunlight, too, are incalculable. As has been discussed, without sunlight, bones cannot get calcified. Sunlight builds the immune system and increases oxygenation of the skin. It brings more blood to the skin surface which helps heal cuts, bruises and rashes. Open wounds and broken bones heal faster in sunlight. Sunlight improves eyesight and hormonal secretions.

But why is sunlight important during exercise? Why is exercising in the open sunshine preferable to indoor exercise?

Before we come to that, let us see why indoor exercise is the poorer choice.

People believe that gymnasia are the most appropriate work out places being equipped with all the mechanical and electronic essentials in fitness management. However gyms prove to be more of a liability to health rather than an advantage. Gyms are often the perfect breeding grounds for noxious germs. In fact instead of getting those dream biceps you could get thoroughly undesirable, relentless infections.

If you fail to take necessary hygiene measures, going to the gym can turn out to be a major health hazard instead of a health benefit. Germs creep up everywhere, right from the exercise equipment you use to the spigot on the drinking water fountain and damp towels. Locker rooms are nothing but 'home-sweet-home' to bacteria and fungi. The constant poor ventilation, warmth and moisture only superadded by the absence of sunlight, render the rooms pathogen-friendly. Locker rooms in gyms are equivalent to what agar culture plates are in labs - media for colonies of bacteria!

You can efficiently prevent the unwanted colds and risks of contracting the dreadful athlete's foot, staphylococcal infections and other gym goers' germs by avoiding these places and embracing the outdoors instead.

In the male physiology, muscular development is linked to the production of the male hormone, testosterone. The old Greek practice of exercising nude on a warm sandy beach was used to develop a healthy muscular body. When sunlight falls on any part of the body, testosterone production increases substantially, but when it strikes the male genitals directly, secretion of the hormone is greatest.

Sunlight exposure has a dramatic impact on testosterone production in males, as plasma testosterone levels decline from November through April, and then rise steadily increase through the spring and summer until they peak in October. This directly impacts reproductive rates, and accordingly, the month of June has the highest rate of conception.

Those living in lower latitudes with generally lower precipitation rates have a year-round advantage in testosterone levels and the corresponding increase in sperm production. Indeed, the Caucasian movement from Europe into lower latitudes was followed by higher birth rates, which were partly due to the sunlight-induced testosterone levels.

A study at Boston State Hospital proved that ultraviolet light increases the level of testosterone by 120% when the chest or back is exposed to sunlight. The hormone, however, increases by a whopping 200% when genital skin is exposed to the sun!

Regular sunbathing increases the strength and size of all muscle groups in the male physique. The combination of sun and exercise is, therefore, ideal to develop a strong and healthy body with optimal reproductive abilities.

There are more than 40 million men in the U.S. suffering from low levels of testosterone. But the vast majority of them don't even know it. As the tremendous popularity of Viagra suggests, many of these men are experiencing symptoms of male sexual dysfunction. Others find themselves fighting more subtle battles against obesity, fatigue, depression and insomnia-common symptoms of low testosterone that most doctors overlook or attribute to the natural process of aging or stress. Testosterone levels reach a peak during a man's early twenties. Aging and lifestyle factors such as stress, improper diet, physical inactivity, smoking, drinking and the use of prescription medications can significantly reduce these levels.

Standard laboratory tests have failed to pinpoint the problem. While medical science has determined that while a man's total (protein-bound) testosterone levels remain relatively stable over time, his bio-available (free) levels gradually decline at an alarming rate of 2% each year beginning at age thirty. This means that a man in his sixties is functioning with only about 40% of the testosterone he had in his twenties. However, when standard laboratory tests are performed, most men typically have only their total levels of testosterone evaluated. Their more important bio-available levels go unchecked.

To make matters worse, most physicians require a diagnosis of hypogonadism (a medical term used to classify total testosterone levels that fall below a specified laboratory limit) prior to prescribing any testosterone replacement medication. As a result, millions of American men who are suffering from symptoms of low testosterone are walking around undiagnosed and untreated.

Adequate exercise helps keep men feeling and looking fit by naturally stimulating testosterone release, and by preventing its breakdown. The duration, intensity and frequency of exercise all determine a man's levels of testosterone. Be aware that testosterone levels increase most with short, periodic, more intense activity. They decrease with prolonged, frequent activity. Studies show testosterone levels increase with 45 to 60 minutes of exercise. After this time, however, testosterone levels begin to decline. Healthy levels of testosterone are necessary for muscle growth and repair. Since frequent, extended training doesn't allow sufficient time for testosterone levels to recover, symptoms of over-training may develop. These symptoms include muscle soreness, diminished performance, fatigue, immune suppression and poor mood.

Guidelines for Increasing Muscle and Maximizing the Effects of Exercise on Testosterone:

- Focus on low-volume, high-intensity strength training.
- Limit your exercise sessions to 60 minutes or less.
- Exercise at high-intensity, no more than 2 or 3 times weekly.
- Do all aerobic exercise (except for warm-ups and cool-downs) on separate days (or at least at separate times during the day) from strength training.
- For optimum fitness, change your exercise regimen every eight to twelve weeks.

Women, of course, benefit from sunlight, too. Their levels of female hormones rise when they are exposed to particularly one specific portion of UV light i.e. 290-340

111

nanometers (UVB), which is assumed to be dangerous and useless.

Women who have only very little exposure to sunlight often suffer from menstrual problems or sometimes, have no menstrual periods at all. They can re-establish a healthy menstrual cycle by sunbathing regularly and spending several hours of the day outdoors. Normalization of the menstrual cycle can occur within a few weeks after starting sunlight therapy.

Infertility is associated with low vitamin D, and PMS can be completely reversed by addition of calcium, magnesium and vitamin D. Vitamin D supports production of estrogen in women. Menstrual migraine is also associated with low levels of vitamin D and calcium.

Given these findings, it may well be that constant lack of sun exposure, along with physical congestion, is the main cause of the increased infertility problems among the city populations in the world.

If you do a little research, you will find that there is a long tradition of associating sunlight and mental and sexual health. The summer solstice, just for example has long be linked with fertility and sexuality around the globe. Whether it is the Maypole Dance or a June Wedding, there is nothing like planting and harvest time to get people to celebrate. The ancient Shamans used the warmer months to practice ancient fertility and sexuality rituals. Yes - summer and the hot sun have been studied by present day scientists all over again, only proving what the ancients already knew - that fertility and sex drive increase when sun shines brighter!

Less sunlight exposure puts our sex drive and fertility rates into slow drive. A decrease in female fertility in winter has long been documented. It has been an often investigated phenomenon even since the North Pole explorer Admiral Byrd's observations a century ago. His expedition reported that Eskimo women lacked menstruation, and thus ovulation, during the periods of 24 hour darkness in their winter.

As of today, the use and interest in light therapy has been widely explored as a treatment for infertility. Research on light therapy has suggested that our decreased exposure to natural sunlight reduces fertility. Apparently, being an office bee does nothing for one's fertility rate. The lighting in an office setting is much of much lower grade and intensity as compared to sunlight and lacks the full spectrum of sunlight. It is hardly any substitute.

Dr. Edmond Dewan John Rock Reproductive Clinic in Boston was among one of the first to use light therapy to treat infertile couples. Couples were given a specially designed light to keep on while they were asleep for three nights a month. The three nights were planned to be the same three days over which ovulation was expected to take place. The couples using the light therapy had a much higher rate of conception than those not using the light.

If you want to improve your sex life or fertility rates, rather than using one of the currently available costly treatments and risking your health due to their serious side effects, I would recommend that you first try the sun.

Sunlight therapy can also help those who suffer from high blood pressure.

Mean blood pressures and the prevalence of hypertension vary in different parts of the world. In general, blood pressures rise at increasing distances from the Equator, and they are higher in winter than in summer. Blood pressures also vary among racial and ethnic groups, with dark-skinned people in the U.S. and the U.K. having a higher prevalence of hypertension than lighter-skinned people of European origin.

A researcher at the University of Alabama hypothesizes that differences in exposure to sunlight and the resulting synthesis of vitamin D may at least partly account for these geographic, seasonal and racial blood pressure differences. Sunlight-induced synthesis of vitamin D decreases with increasing distance from the Equator, and it is lower in winter than in summer. People with deeply pigmented skin

113

synthesize less vitamin D than light-skinned people do when exposed to the same amount of sunlight. Differences in vitamin D synthesis influence parathyroid hormone status, which in turn may alter blood pressure.

The same researcher notes that geographic and racial differences in blood pressure and the prevalence of hypertension have usually been related to dietary changes, particularly sodium and potassium consumption, to intrinsic genetic differences in renal hemodynamics and sodium metabolism, and to the social and economic stresses of industrialization and modern living. The new hypothesis complements rather than replaces these explanations. The hypothesis that ultraviolet-induced vitamin D synthesis affects blood pressure could be tested by exposing salt-sensitive, low-renin hypertensive Europeans and Africans to varying doses of light or perhaps, more easily, by supplementing them with vitamin D.

Another study, conducted by scientists at Bologna University, Italy, of several tribes across central Asia, living at heights from 600m to 3,200m above sea level, produced evidence that confirmed the inverse relationship between sunlight and blood pressure. Hypertension was much more frequent at low altitudes than at high altitude. The strength of UVB, the wavelength that produces vitamin D in the skin, is much greater when the atmosphere is thinner.

Several independent studies have demonstrated that hypertensive patients who followed a vigorous exercise program for 6 months lowered their blood pressure by 15%, whereas those who had one single exposure to the ultraviolet light of the sun had markedly lower blood pressure readings for 5 to 6 days. Exercising in the sun could, therefore, be one of the best non-medical treatments for hypertension, cost-free and without any side effects.

One of the biggest lies in medicine is that a person must stay on hypertensive drugs for a lifetime if he/she is hypertensive. It is simply not true. In most people, sunlight and a plant-based nutrition program can easily bring blood pressure levels to normal. Ask your physician before changing any prescribed medication, of course.

At the same time, both exercise and sunbathing increase the heart's efficiency, which is measured by the amount of blood pumped by the heart at each beat. A single exposure to the ultraviolet rays of the sun increases heart efficiency by an average of 39%, again lasting for as long as 5 to 6 days. Such an approach could effectively replace drugs currently used to stimulate the heart.

It should be noted that sunlight does not act like a drug that merely suppresses the symptoms of disease but rather restores balance in body and mind. Sunlight should more so be recognized as a necessary nutrient than a miracle medicine. Diabetics, too, can benefit from exercise and sunlight.

The study by Dr Chantal Mathieu of the University of Leuven, Belgium, and other researchers found that low levels of the vitamin D could be linked to the development of autoimmune disorders such as diabetes and thyroid diseases.

Sunlight, which is a major source of vitamin D, appears to lower type 1 diabetes risk for children. This discovery was recently made at the University of San Diego Moores Cancer Center.

Type 1 Diabetes is the second most common chronic childhood disease, behind asthma. About 1.5 million Americans have type 1 Diabetes, and about 15,000 new cases are diagnosed each year. The disease is the main cause of blindness in young and middle-aged adults and is among the leading causes of kidney failure and transplants in that age group, according to a news release about the study.

According to the study, children living near the equator, which has a high abundance of sun light, are far less likely to develop type 1 diabetes than those living at more northerly or southerly points, which have much less sunlight. According to study, author Dr. Cedric Garland, higher serum levels of vitamin D are associated with reduced incidence rates of type 1 diabetes worldwide.

By plotting the location (using latitude, with zero being the equator, negative being the southern hemisphere, and positive being the northern hemisphere) on the horizontal axis, versus type 1 diabetes incidence on the vertical axis, a parabola resulted. The parabolic association is strong and distinctive. 51 regions were accounted for. This association was present regardless of a locations economic and health care status, meaning that even poorer countries near the equator, with less developed healthcare systems, had a lower type 1 diabetes incidence rate.

Careful control over the amount of food and drink that formerly sedentary, overweight people ingest during and after short-term exercise has a significant impact on insulin action. The same study showed a measurable effect on the subjects' cardiovascular disease (CVD) risk factors, according to researchers in the Exercise Science Department at the University of Massachusetts, Amherst. After only 6 days of enough treadmill exercise to burn 500 kilocalories (k/cal) each day, the 8 subjects in the negative energy balance (NEG) group, who received no energy replacement, showed a significant (p=0.037) 40% increase in insulin action (measured by glucose rate of disappearance/steady state insulin). However insulin action was unchanged in the zero energy balance group (ZERO group) which was required to finish a sports drink during exercise and additional food afterwards to 'replace' the 500 k/cal.

The same subjects showed positive trends in both traditional and novel CVD risk factors, though not at a significant level. On the other hand, the subjects in the ZERO group showed either virtually no change or bad changes in CVD risk factors.

The blood sugar levels of diabetics drop when they exercise or sunbathe. A single exposure to sunlight stimulates the production of the enzyme phosphorylase, which decreases the amount of stored glycogen. Two hours after sun exposure, another enzyme, glycogen synthesize, increases storage of glycogen in the tissues, while lowering blood sugar levels. Thus, sunlight acts just like insulin. The effect may last for days. It is important for diabetics to know that they may need to adjust their insulin dose and should, therefore, regularly consult their doctor while gradually increasing their body's exposure to sunlight.

Furthermore, both sunlight and exercise have beneficial effects on reducing stress levels. These include a decrease of nervousness, anxiety, and emotional imbalance, an increase of stress tolerance, self confidence, imagination, and creativity, positive changes in personality and moods, and a reduction of unhealthy habits such as cigarette smoking and alcoholism.

Vitamin D is an important nutrient and is necessary to health - both physical and emotional. Because vitamin D is thought to benefit the body and enhance the mood, natural sunlight can be linked to stress relief. The serotonin levels, the chemical responsible for mood elevation in the brain, are increased in the presence of the sun. As a result, better and more positive moods can result from being outdoors during daytime hours.

Artificial sunlight is used as a treatment for depression called 'light therapy'. Light therapy may be achieved with the use of a light box that mimics the effects of natural sunlight. This therapy is thought to improve your mood by causing biochemical changes to occur, thus relieving symptoms of depression. Another common practice to gain the benefits of vitamin D is sun tanning. Many individuals claim that tanning aids in stress reduction and relaxation.

Sunlight is beneficial in virtually each and every health issue which may arise from the disturbances in any of the three spheres of human expression - physical, mental or spiritual. It is useful in cases varying from commonplace functional derangements and emotional turbulence to gross organic disorders with abnormal tissue structural changes. Studies from Russia even show that duodenal ulcers greatly improve through regular exposure to the sun.

American research found that when exposure to sunlight was added to fitness programs, subjects had a 19 % increase in performance as measured by physical fitness tests.

In the past, vitamin D has been shown to maintain calcium homeostasis and improve bone density, lowering the risk of fractures. Results of a published survey suggest vitamin D bolsters muscle strength and function, therefore decreasing the chance for falls that may lead to fractures.

Researchers examined the relationship between vitamin D levels and muscle strength and function in 4,100 subjects, about half men and half women, age 60 and older, with the mean age being about 71. Vitamin D concentrations were measured in all participants, who were then classified into 5 groups, or quintiles, according to their vitamin D level. Participants also were classified by activity level. About 75 % of them were active, meaning they had walked one mile without stopping, swam, jogged, bicycled, danced, exercised or gardened in the previous month. Those that had not, about one in four, were considered inactive. Researchers also controlled for calcium intake, sex, age, race or ethnicity.

Using a timed 8-foot walk test and a repeated sit-to-stand test, investigators assessed each subject's lower extremity functionality. Those who performed the tests in a shorter amount of time were judged as having better muscle strength and functionality.

Subjects in the highest quintile of vitamin D concentration had a mean 5 % decrease in time of 0.27 second in the 8-foot walk test compared to those in the lowest quintile. For the sit-to-stand test the highest quintile of participants had a mean 3.9 % decrease of 0.67 seconds compared to the lowest group.

Therefore, researchers associated higher vitamin D concentration with improved lower extremity function. The best results were seen in subjects with levels from 22.5 to 40 nmol/L. Positive results were also seen in the 40-90 nmol/L range.

118

Researchers summarized that in both active and inactive subjects, those with higher concentrations have better musculoskeletal function. They noted that while concentrations of 40 nmol/L or greater are desirable for optimal function, concentrations as high as 100 nmol/L appear advantageous.

They went on to conclude that vitamin D supplementation may offer a way to improve lower-extremity function in both active and inactive elderly subjects.

Studies have proved that persons exposed to UV light had 50 % fewer incidences of colds than those who weren't. Their immune systems were maintained at a high level of efficiency.

Also, children who received extra UV light during wintertime had a marked increase in physical fitness.

Taking a vacation to a sunny locale, for example, can help balance the immune system during wintertime.

Spending some time outside every day, even if it is cold, also helps to fill one's UV requirements. UV lamps can also be very useful. The UV Lamp Module sold on Dr. Mercola's website, www.mercola.com, produces hydroxyl radicals and other elements that neutralize toxins and effectively destroy microbes up to .001 microns that come in contact with its powerful UV-C rays. And if you are on pain medication, check this out: A recent hospital study found that patients in sunnier rooms needed fewer painkillers than patients in darker rooms. In fact, they were able to cut their drug costs by 21%.

Chapter 13:
What Makes the Sun so "Dangerous" – The Fat Connection!

Sunlight is optimally beneficial for those who eat a balanced diet according to their individual requirements and body type.

The human body requires food to provide energy for all life process and for growth, repair and maintenance of cells and tissues. The dietetic needs vary according to age, sex and occupation. A balanced diet is one that contains different types of foods in such quantities and proportions that the need for calories, minerals, vitamins and other nutrients is adequately met and small provision is made for extra nutrients to withstand short durations of leanness. Eating a well balanced diet on a regular basis and staying at your ideal weight are critical factors in maintaining your emotional and physical wellbeing.

Fluid intake in the form of water based drinks is also essential for good health. Water is essential for the correct functioning of the kidneys and bowels.

A poor diet laden with fats and processed foods can predispose a person to sunburn or other damage. Sunbathing is dangerous, yes, but only for those who are on a standard, high fat American diet or do not get an abundance of vegetables, whole grains and fresh fruits.

At the end of a two year study, skin cancer patients on a low fat diet had significantly fewer lesions than those who had not changed their diet.

The heliotherapists of the previous century placed great emphasis on diet to maximize the sun's benefits. Even Dr. Rollier insisted that healthful meals were an integral part of treatment, suggesting that well nourished skin responds better to sunlight that mineral deficient skin.

A good diet is of such profound importance that sunbathing can even prove to be downright hazardous for those who live on a diet rich in acid-forming, highly processed foods and refined fats or products made with them - basically foods that are not created by nature - unnatural foods. Alcohol, cigarettes, and other mineral and vitamin depleting substances, such as allopathic and hallucinogenic drugs, can also make the skin highly vulnerable to UV radiation.

The need to laboriously process food into artificial low-nutrition 'junk' is a mystery. Human beings, globally, seem to be choosing easier ways out in all conceivable walks of life. Lassitude defines our actions - or rather the lack of them. The new age comforts and conveniences are nothing but licenses to laziness, and yet we choose to waste time and energy on thoroughly unnecessary useless complex procedures to 'refine/process/reduce' food that is naturally available (in an entirely wholesome form) into something unhealthy. Why does man want to take the trouble to make trouble for his own self?

Continual associations between increasing skin cancer risk and diets that are high in protein, animal fats, junk foods, soft drinks, vegetable oils, hydrogenated oils, animal and vegetable shortenings, and dairy products (trouble foods) are being recorded. Eating a high fat diet and spending lots of time in the sun is a bad combination.

Our bodies are not only exposed to unhealthy oils in food alone. You can also find the foul fuel in skin care products such as suntan oils and skin lotions. Unhealthy oils in skin care products can also damage your skin. The danger lies in the fact that UV rays react with fats in the body to form 'free radicals'. These products are damaging and can lead to cancerous transformations of the otherwise normal cells.

Although with this new revelation, one may understand the sun to be the hazardous influence here, but the fact is that the real culprit is a diet more or less full of fat and free of fresh nutrients and antioxidants. It is the dietary indiscretion that sends the defaulter to the guillotine and orders the execution. Sunlight is only a modality in the system.

121

If you eat a diet high in fruits, vegetables, and whole grains, you would be getting plenty of nutrients, antioxidants, and other plant substances that will help prevent the formation of the fearsome free radicals. Fresh, plant foods facilitate and appropriately energize your body so as to be able to handle exposure to sunlight. Antioxidants protect your skin from burning too quickly. They also prevent premature aging.

Apart from the objectionable dietetic habits, several modern medications are responsible for turning the sun from friend to foe.

Medications can render skin abnormally sensitive to sunlight, what can be referred to as 'drug-induced photosensitivity'. Many of these drugs are commonly used including most of the tetracycline antibiotics, birth control pills, antihistamines, antidepressants and many retinoids (such as Vitamin A derivatives).

Drug-induced photosensitivity refers to the development of cutaneous disease as a result of the combined effects of a chemical and light. Exposure to either the chemical or the light alone is not sufficient to induce the disease. However, when photo-activation of the chemical occurs, one or more cutaneous manifestations may arise. These include phototoxic and photo-allergic reactions, a planus lichenoides reaction, pseudoporphyria, and subacute cutaneous lupus erythematosus. Photosensitivity reactions may result from systemic medications or topically applied compounds.

Wavelengths within the UVA (320-400 nm) range and, for certain compounds, within the visible range, are more likely to cause drug-induced photosensitivity reactions, although occasionally UVB (290-320 nm) can also be responsible for such effects.

Phototoxic reactions occur because of the damaging effects of light-activated compounds on cell membranes and, in some instances, DNA. By contrast, photo-allergic reactions are cell-mediated immune responses to a light-activated compound. Phototoxic reactions develop in most

122

individuals if they are exposed to sufficient amounts of light and drug. Typically, they appear as an exaggerated sunburn response. Photo-allergic reactions resemble allergic contact dermatitis, with a distribution limited to sun-exposed areas of the body. However, when the reactions are severe or prolonged, they may extend into covered areas of skin.

Photo-allergic reactions develop in only a minority of individuals exposed to the compound and light. They are less prevalent than phototoxic skin reactions. The amount of drug required to elicit photo-allergic reactions is considerably smaller than that required for phototoxic reactions. Moreover, photo-allergic reactions are a form of cell-mediated immunity. Their onset often is delayed by as long as 24-72 hours after exposure to the drug and light. By contrast, phototoxic responses often occur within minutes or hours of light exposure.

Phototoxic reactions are considerably more common than photo-allergic reactions.

400 drugs are known to cause light sensitive and photo-allergic reactions. If you are not sure whether any of your medications are likely to cause photosensitivity, check with your doctor or pharmacist.

Both phototoxic and photo allergic reactions occur in sun-exposed areas of skin, including the face, V of the neck, and dorsa of the hands and forearms. The hair-bearing scalp, post-auricular and periorbital areas, and submental portion of the chin are usually spared. A widespread eruption suggests exposure to a systemic photosensitizer, whereas a localized eruption indicates a reaction to a locally applied topical photosensitizer.

Phototoxic reactions in skin can appear as follows:-

• Acute photo-toxicity often begins as an exaggerated sunburn reaction with erythema and edema that occurs within minutes to hours of light exposure. Vesicles and bullae may develop with severe reactions. The lesions often heal with hyperpigmentation, which resolves in a matter of weeks to months. Chronic phototoxicity may also appear as an exaggerated sunburn reaction.

• Other less common skin manifestations of phototoxicity include pigmentary changes. A blue-gray pigmentation is associated with several agents, including amiodarone, chlorpromazine, and some tricyclic antidepressants. Reactions to psoralen-containing botanicals (phytophotodermatitis) and drugs may resolve, with a brownish discoloration. Frequently, the pigmentary change is preceded by a typical sunburn reaction. If the reaction is not severe, some patients may not notice the erythema.

• Photosensitizing drugs may also cause a lichen planus-like eruption in sun-exposed areas. Drugs likely to cause this type of reaction include demeclocycline, hydrochlorothiazide, enalapril, quinine, quinidine, chloroquine, and hydroxychloroquine.

• Pseudoporphyria, which involves porphyria cutanea tarda-like changes of skin fragility and subepidermal blisters on the dorsa of hands, may occur after exposure to naproxen, nalidixic acid, tetracycline, sulfonylureas, furosemide, dapsone, amiodarone, bumetanide, and pyridoxine. Frequent use of sun-tanning beds and chronic renal failure are other predisposing factors.

Phototoxic reactions in nails:-
Photo-onycholysis, or separation of the distal nail plate from the nail bed, is another manifestation. Photo-onycholysis has been reported with the use of many systemic medications, including tetracycline, psoralen, chloramphenicol, fluoroquinolones, oral contraceptives, quinine, and mercaptopurine. Photo-onycholysis may be the only manifestation of phototoxicity in individuals with heavily pigmented skin.

Photoallergic reactions in skin appear as follows:-
• Photoallergic reactions typically develop in sensitized individuals 24-48 hours after exposure. The reaction usually

manifests as a pruritic eczematous eruption. Erythema and vesiculation are present in the acute phase.

• More chronic exposure results in erythema, lichenification, and scaling.

• Hyperpigmentation does not occur in photoallergic reactions.

Coming back to dietary misdemeanors, let us understand what the most dangerous foods are. In particular, polyunsaturated fats as contained in refined and vitamin E depleted products, such as thin vegetable oil, mayonnaise, salad dressings, and most brands of margarine, pose a specifically high risk in the development of skin cancer and most other cancers.

Studies have even linked high intakes of total fat to increased risk of redeveloping a squamous cell carcinoma among people who have a history of skin cancer.

In addition to protecting the skin from too much sunlight, people who have a history of skin cancer would benefit from lowering their total fat intake.

Ibiebele and colleagues studied the diets of 457 men and 600 women, who were 25 to 75 years old. They determined their daily intake of saturated, monounsaturated and polyunsaturated fats in meats, fried foods, on breads and vegetables, and in cooking. The men and women lived in the sub-tropical area of Nambour, Queensland, an area with high concentration of ultraviolet sunlight, the researchers reported in the International Journal of Cancer. During the follow up lasting 11 years, 267 of the study participants developed 664 basal cell skin tumors. Another 127 men and women developed a total of 235 squamous cell skin tumors. In the subjects with a prior history of skin cancer, higher total fat intake was associated with about a twofold increased risk of squamous cell cancer of the skin. This finding, the investigators noted, "supports the body of literature, which shows that people with prior skin cancer do not benefit from a high fat diet".

Since 1974, the increase of polyunsaturated fats has been the blame for the alarming increase in malignant melanoma in Australia. We are all told that the sun causes it. Are Australians going out in the sun any more now than they were 50 years ago? Not at all! What they are certainly doing is eating more polyunsaturated oils. Victims of the disease have been found to have polyunsaturated oils in their skin cells. Polyunsaturated oils are oxidized readily by ultra-violet radiation from the sun and form those harmful free radicals and can proceed to damage the cell's DNA and then lead to the deregulation we call cancer. Saturated fats are, on the other hand, stable. They do not oxidize and form free radicals.

Untreated, expeller-pressed[6] oils contain both types of fats, with varying ratios. Both kinds of fat are useful for the body. Sesame oil, for example has 50% polyunsaturated fats and 50% monounsaturated fats. If the monounsaturated fats are removed from the oil through the refining process, its polyunsaturated fats become highly reactive and damaging to cells. This phenomenon is quite easy to understand. Polyunsaturated fats are more vulnerable to lipid peroxidation (rancidity) than monounsaturated fats. In other words, they rapidly attract a large number of oxygen free radicals and become oxidized. Oxygen radicals are generated when oxygen molecules lose an electron. This makes them highly reactive. These free radicals may quickly attack and damage cells, tissues, and organs. They can be formed in refined, polyunsaturated fats when these are exposed to sunlight before consumption. Free radicals may also form in the tissues after the oil has been eaten.

Oxygen is essential for life yet it is also inherently dangerous to our existence. This is referred to as the oxygen paradox.

Oxygen is required in the normal metabolism within the cell to create energy (called oxidation) and in the process

---

[6] One of the methods employed for the extraction of edible oils, explained in the next chapter

active free oxygen radicals are created. We produce free radicals with every breath we take. Consuming polyunsaturated oils only increases the load of free radicals in the body.

Free radicals are the things that cause cut apples and potatoes to turn brown. They are also the cause of fatty meats turning rancid.

Free radicals are incomplete, unstable molecules. Molecules of oxygen, fatty acids, and amino acids are the basic building blocks in nature. Electrons hold molecules together and normal molecules have pairs of electrons. When the molecule loses 1 electron it becomes a free radical. It is unbalanced and is extremely reactive with other molecules.

In order to regain their missing electrons, they steal electrons from other molecules wherever they can and the deprived victim molecules get damaged in the process and become free radicals themselves. The stealing of electrons is a chain reaction. If they are not rapidly neutralized by an antioxidant they may create even more volatile free radicals or cause damage to the cell membranes, vessel walls, proteins, fats or even the DNA nuclei of the cells. Cell damage by free radicals is called oxidative stress. Scientific research has established that the root cause of more than 70 chronic degenerative diseases is due to oxidative stress, or cell damage by free radicals.

Free radicals can burst through cell walls and alter the DNA, thus causing the cell to malfunction.

Oxidative stress has the potential to overpower all of our protective systems and cause chronic degenerative diseases. When the damaged proteins, fats, cell membranes, and DNA structures are not properly repaired, they can create further problems in cell function. The mutations caused in the nucleus can result in cancer.

Damaged lipids lead to rigid cell membranes. Oxidized cholesterol often leads to hardening of the arteries and poorly repaired DNA chains lead to cell mutation (future generation of cells) as implicated in cancer and aging.

127

As time goes on, our immune systems gradually lose vigor in their response to diseases and infection. So it is of prime importance that we make every effort to avoid a free radical overdose from overuse or overconsumption of the fats and oils that produce them.

Before we go any further, I believe that it is important to know that all fats are NOT the same. A common misconception the general public and some ignorant nutritionists hold is that all fats are essentially the same. This is not true. There are, to be sure, certain fats and oils that we need to avoid, but one must always be very specific as to what those are. Let us define our terms to end the confusion once and for all.

Fatty acids are chains of carbon and hydrogen atoms linked together in certain ways with an acid, or carboxyl group, attached to their end. When three fatty acids are bonded together with a glycerol molecule, the result is a triglyceride.

In lipid biochemistry, all fatty acids are classified according to the number of carbon atoms present in their structure, as well as the degree of saturation, or how many hydrogen atoms are bonded to the carbons. A fatty acid that has two hydrogen atoms linked up to each carbon atom is saturated. A fatty acid with two hydrogen atoms missing is monounsaturated and a fatty acid with four or more hydrogen atoms missing is polyunsaturated.

All fats and oils, whether of animal or vegetable origin, are blends of these three types, but with one usually predominating, depending on the food in question.

Saturated fats predominate principally in animal fats, though palm and coconut oils are noted plant sources. Monounsaturated fats abound in nuts, avocadoes, olive oil, and some animal fats (especially lard). Polyunsaturated fats (PUFAs) mostly make up vegetable oils, but significant amounts are found in fish oils and chicken skin.

The more a fat is saturated, the more stable it is chemically. Saturated and monounsaturated fats do not go rancid easily if stored properly. Likewise, these fats are more stable under heat, making them ideal for cooking. Polyunsaturated fats, however, especially those of vegetable origin, are not as stable and go rancid more quickly, even in the body. Polyunsaturated oils are so vulnerable that even at room temperature and in subdued light, oxidation occurs inside the bottle. All polyunsaturated vegetable oils sold at grocery stores have become rancid to some degree before you even bring them home. Because the oils have been highly refined and deodorized you cannot smell or taste anything, but the free radicals are there, waiting to attack your body.

If you store the oil in the cupboard at room temperature, the oxidation process continues. When you open the bottle and expose the oil to oxygen in the air, oxidation is accelerated. If you leave it out on the counter where it is exposed to light, oxidation progresses even faster. To make matters worse, if you use the oil in cooking you greatly accelerate the rate of oxidation and free radical formation. For this reason, you should never use polyunsaturated oils in cooking. Most people do this all the time. They buy a bottle of soybean oil for instance, and keep it in the cupboard for months together and use it along with margarine for all their cooking. . Eating a hamburger and French fries can flood your body with free radicals. Both foods are heated with refined oils. The heating process that the oils in these foods undergo greatly increases their oxidation and, therefore, tissue-damaging effects. It is no wonder why cancer, diabetes, Alzheimer's and other diseases associated with free radicals are becoming more and more prevalent nowadays. One of the best ways to prevent these diseases is to not use polyunsaturated oils in cooking.

The polyunsaturated fats in refined oils (stripped of their monounsaturated fats), are virtually indigestible and thereby become dangerous to the body. Margarine, for example, is just one molecule away from plastic, and therefore extremely difficult to digest.

Originally margarines were made of beef suet, milk and water. Later the recipes changed to include lard, whale oil and the oils of olive, coconut, ground nut and cottonseed. By the middle of the 20th-century, an emulsion of soya bean and water was substituted for milk. Margarines could then be made entirely of inexpensive oils from vegetable sources. In all these forms, margarine was the poor relation to butter.

In the 1920s a new disease had suddenly 'taken off' all over the industrialized world. By the 1940s it had become a leading cause of premature death - and nobody knew why. In 1950, an American scientist hypothesized that cholesterol might be to blame. In 1953, another American, Ancel Keys, compared levels of this disease in seven countries with the amounts of fat in those countries. And so was born the 'Diet-Heart' hypothesis. The new disease was coronary heart disease.

To reduce the risk of a heart attack, Ancel Keys recommended cutting down on the vegetable oils and margarines. However, it was discovered that vegetable oils, which are composed largely of unsaturated fats and oils, tended to lower blood cholesterol levels, while saturated fats tended to raise them. And by that time, it had been decided, largely by majority vote, that raised cholesterol increased the risk of a heart attack. Cholesterol had become the big culprit. With the advent of the 'Prudent Diet' in the U.S.A. in 1982, and COMA's introduction of 'healthy eating' in Britain two years later, the fats in our diet changed even more dramatically: we were told to avoid animal fats such as butter and lard, which have a larger proportion of saturated fats, and to favor largely polyunsaturated vegetable margarines and cooking oils. Now margarines could be priced to rival butter. Recently, margarines have been developed specifically to lower cholesterol levels, and prices have risen again. Benecol, for example, made from tree bark is considerably more expensive than butter.

Is margarine really a natural food?

The polyunsaturated fats used to make margarine are generally obtained from vegetable sources: sunflower seed, cottonseed, and soybean. As such they might be thought of as natural foods. Usually, however, they are forced onto the public in the form of highly processed margarines, spreads and oils and, as such, they are anything but natural.

In 1989, the petroleum-based solvent, benzene, that is known to cause cancer, was found in Perrier mineral water at a mean concentration of 14 parts per billion. This was enough to cause Perrier to be removed from supermarket shelves. The first process in the manufacture of margarine is the extraction of the oils from the seeds, and this is usually done using similar petroleum-based solvents. Although these are then boiled off, this stage of the process still leaves about 10 parts per million of the solvents in the product. That is 700 times as much as 14 parts per billion.

The oils then go through more than ten other processes: degumming, bleaching, hydrogenation, neutralization, fractionation, deodorisation, emulsification, inter-esterification, etc. that include heat treatment at 140-160C with a solution of caustic soda; the use of nickel, a metal that is known to cause cancer, as a catalyst, with up to 50 parts per million of the nickel left in the product; the addition of antioxidants such as butylated hydroxyanisol (E320). These antioxidants are again usually petroleum based and are widely believed to cause cancer.

The hydrogenation process, that solidifies the oils so that they are spreadable, produces trans-fatty acids that rarely occur in nature.

The heat treatment alone is enough to render these margarines nutritionally inadequate. When the massive chemical treatment and unnatural fats are added, the end product can hardly be called either natural or healthy.

You may be interested in a list of the ingredients that are generally present in butter and margarine:

Butter: milk, fat (cream), a little salt.

Margarine: Edible oils, edible fats, salt or potassium chloride, ascorbyl palmitate, butylated hydroxyanisole, phospholipids, tert-butylhydroquinone, mono- and di-glycerides of fat-forming fatty acids, disodium guanylate, diacetyltartaric and fatty acid esters of glycerol, Propyl, octyl or dodecyl gallate (or mixtures thereof), tocopherols, propylene glycol mono- and di-esters, sucrose esters of fatty acids, curcumin, annatto extracts, tartaric acid, 3,5,trimethylhexanal, ß-apo-carotenoic acid methyl or ethyl ester, skim milk powder, xanthophylls, canthaxanthin, vitamins A and D.

It is obvious that polyunsaturated oils and highly refined oils are best avoided while the healthier mono saturated and saturated oils are by far the more preferable choices.

Olive oil is all right to use because it is primarily a monounsaturated fat and, therefore, much more stable than polyunsaturated oils. It is of great use mostly for salads and low temperature foods. It is good to store it in the refrigerator and to use it up within a month or so.

The only fats you should use for moderate to high temperature cooking are saturated fats like lard, butter, and coconut oil. They contain large quantities of natural antioxidants, which make them much safer against oxidation by free radicals. They are also digested quite easily. Lard has a high smoking point so it makes for good high temperature cooking oil. Coconut oil has the highest content of saturated fat so it serves as an excellent all-purpose cooking oil. It is very stable under heat, but has a relatively low smoking point.

There are many vital nutrients and substances found in saturated fats. Butter, for example, is rich in several trace minerals, including selenium, a key antioxidant and cancer preventer. Several studies have linked low selenium levels with higher cancer and heart disease rates. Butter also contains all the fat-soluble vitamins, especially vitamins A and D, both antioxidants are protective against cancer. In addition it contains fair amounts of two fatty acids: butyric and lauric. Both of these are antifungal, antibacterial, and anticarcinogenic substances. (Coconut and palm kernel oils, and Roquefort cheese are other significant sources of lauric acid.) Butter is also the best source of a particular fatty acid getting a lot of attention lately: conjugated linoleic acid.[7]

Coconut oil is another good example. Formerly used widely in baked goods, this oil is very rich in lauric acid. This fatty acid converts in the intestines into monolaurin, a powerful antifungal, antiviral, and antibacterial substance. Coconut oil also contains caprylic acid, also a powerful antifungal. Recent research shows coconut oil to be stimulatory to the immune system and to offer substantial benefits to HIV+ individuals. Yet these properties are lost amidst a plethora of unwarranted warnings about 'the dangers of saturated fat.'

After learning about the subtle dangers of the unsaturated fats, with a view to escape the trouble, one may want to evade these fats completely. All plants contain unsaturated fats. Even commercial meat has these fats (30% or more) because commercial animals are fed soybeans and corn, both high in unsaturated fats.

Since all plants contain unsaturated oils except fruits and fruit juices, it is impossible to avoid them. However it would be well to remember that the fiber in plants offers a certain

---

[7] Conjugated Linoleic Acid (CLA) is a fatty acid produced by ruminating animals such as cows. It is an isomer of linoleic acid. The natural forms are found in milk fat (especially high fat cheeses) and meat fat. CLA has been shown to inhibit the development of cancer, including breast cancer. The October 2000 issue of the *Journal of the American College of Nutrition* contained a research abstract describing how CLA inhibited breast cancer cell growth. As a side benefit, several studies have shown CLA to promote muscle growth and fat burning by the body. In other words, CLA is a fatty acid that helps you lose unwanted fat and build a leaner body.

Where do you find CLA? Some supplement companies now manufacture CLA in capsule form, but the best source is fat from grass-fed cows. It's important that you look for full fat butter. Why? -Because cows manufacture CLA from grass in their stomachs. Commercially-raised cows which only eat soybeans or corn meal produce little, if any, CLA.

protection against the toxicity from the effects of the chemical resolution of these oils in the body. The polyunsaturated fats in refined oils are difficult to digest, since they are deprived of their natural bulk and are no longer protected against free radicals by their natural protector, vitamin E, a powerful antioxidant (vitamin E interferes with the oxidation process). Vitamin E and many other valuable nutrients are filtered out or destroyed during the refining process.

Some polyunsaturated fats are in fact needed by the body, the so-called essential fatty acids (EFAs).

The two EFAs are linolenic (an omega 3 fatty acid) and linoleic (an omega 6 fatty acid). The '3' and '6' indicate where the first double bond occurs in the fatty acid molecule. For example, in an omega-3 fatty acid, the first double bond occurs at the third carbon atom. The body takes the EFAs and creates other omega-3 and -6 fatty acids and the hormone-like substances called prostaglandins to carry out a host of metabolic functions. In times past, humans consumed a balance of linolenic and other omega-3 fatty acids (found principally in Chia seeds, in cold water fish, walnuts, eggs, flax oil, dark green leafy vegetables, cod liver oil, and some whole grains) and linoleic and other omega-6 fatty acids (found principally in vegetables), and this is as it should be as both are equally important. These fats should not be taken in excess due to the probability of toxic effects. Also, humans and animals have desaturase enzymes, which can synthesize unsaturated fats from oleic and palmitoleic acids when deprived of the so-called essential fatty acids.

The truth is no one has ever given correct physiological evidence that these PUFAs are, in fact, essential components of our 'diet'. They are however, required in small quantities in the body for certain function. During the last 10 years many journal articles have interestingly reported that the body can make its own brand of unsaturated oils in people who do not eat the exogenous ones. Externally obtained PUFAs in bulk overburden and quite merely poison the enzymes inside your body that are necessary for the natural synthesis of unsaturated oils.

Dr. Enig, a well known nutritionist, said that the fats that humans have consumed for millennia were almost always more saturated than unsaturated. It was the easily extractable fat or oil, such as the fat that came from the animal or, in tropical areas, the oil that came from the coconut or palm fruit that was used in cooking. People really didn't have the ability to extract oil from vegetables like corn as they do today. However, people got their EFAs from many of these plants when they were included in the foods the people were eating. This was the way the EFAs were historically consumed. In other words, like our ancestors, it's best to have more saturated fats in our diet and to get your EFAs from whole foods rather than from processed vegetable oils.

Won't increasing your saturated fat intake increase your chances for heart disease, you may wonder. Dr. Enig says it is not so. The idea that dietary saturated fats and cholesterol cause heart disease or 'clogged arteries' is completely wrong. Studies have actually revealed that arterial plaque is mostly made up of unsaturated fats, particularly polyunsaturates."

In fact, the body needs saturated fats in order to properly utilize EFAs. Saturated fats also lower the blood levels of the artery-damaging lipoprotein A (LpA levels are elevated by TFAs-trans fatty acids) and are needed for proper calcium utilization in the bones. They also stimulate the immune system. They are the preferred food for the heart and other vital organs and, along with cholesterol, add structural stability to the cell wall. Dr. Enig further comments: "Increasing one's intake of saturates spares the body's supply of antioxidants which get rapidly used up with a high polyunsaturated fat diet. This is another way by which saturates effectively protect against cancer."

When there is an overabundance of linoleic acid in the diet, however, our body's ability to absorb and utilize linolenic acid is inhibited. This causes a host of undesirable reactions including sexual and immune dysfunction, and increased cancer risk. The Western world has greatly increased its linoleic acid intake due to its higher use of vegetable oils over the past 60 years. Not surprisingly, cancer (and heart disease) rates have skyrocketed.

There is yet another type of 'fatty acid' that is produced during chemical processing called a trans-fatty acid (TFA) . These are unnatural fats that our bodies cannot utilize properly due to their bizarre chemical structure. In a TFA, a liquid vegetable oil has been made solid by forcing hydrogen atoms into it with the help of a nickel catalyst. The hydrogenation process used by the oils and fats industry produces trans-fats, which are more damaging than any other oils and fats because it employs: 1) high heat, 2) a metal catalyst such as nickel, zinc, copper, or other reactive metals, and 3) hydrogen gas. In terms of visual appearance, a hydrogenated fat looks like a saturated one since both are solid at room temperature. This is a volatile combination designed to extract and process oils, but it results in an extremely toxic product that the body reacts to it like it does to other toxins and poisons. Not only are these fats toxic, increasing the body's need for vitamin E and other antioxidants (substances that guard the body against harmful effects), but they also severely depress the immune system. Although these fats and oils are solid and stabilized through the refining, on a molecular level, the TFAs are quite different, making them unusable by the body. Basically the chemical addition of hydrogen to saturate the double bonds causes the oil to become solid, to mimic butter, but that is not all there is to it. These unnatural oils are harmful in innumerable ways. A Welsh study linked the concentration of these artificial trans-fats in body fat with high rates of death from heart disease.

The Dutch government has already banned any products containing trans-fatty acids. Some of the undesirable consequences are as mentioned below:

- Increases LDL-cholesterol– the bad type of cholesterol that causes plaque deposits in the arteries and ultimately increases risk of cardiovascular disease. Research at Harvard Medical School, in which the dietary habits of 85,000 women were observed for over 8 years, found that those eating margarine had an increased risk of coronary heart disease. Further studies have shown that trans-fatty acids prevent the body from processing Low Density Lipoprotein (LDL) or bad cholesterol, thereby raising blood cholesterol to abnormal levels.
- Trans-fat consumption also reduces the particle size of the LDL molecules, making them more damaging to the arteries.
- Decreases HDL-cholesterol – the good type of cholesterol.
- Promotes the inflammatory response – this is an overstimulation of the immune system that has been implicated in heart disease, stroke, diabetes, and other chronic conditions.
- May increase the risk of diabetes - there is scientific evidence which suggests that trans fat consumption can lead to insulin resistance and ultimately increase your risk of developing type 2 diabetes.
- Trans-fats inhibit the cell's ability to use oxygen, which is required to burn foodstuffs to carbon dioxide and water. Cells, which are inhibited in completing their metabolic processes, may thus become cancerous.
- The trans-fats also make the blood thicker by increasing the stickiness of the platelets. This multiplies the chances of blood clots and the buildup of fatty deposits, which can lead to heart disease.

These fake fats can be obtained from vegetable fats and oils derived from plants such as canola oil (from rape seed), soy, safflower, sunflower, soybean, and corn. They can also be found in products that contain these fats, such as margarine, salad dressing, mayonnaise, cooking and baking oils and fats, and many processed and prepared foods that contain these fats and oils. Margarine can contain up to 54 % of them, vegetable shortening up to 58 %. Some typical products that contain these plastic oils and fats are breads, pastries, cake, cookies, muffins, buns, French fries, potato chips, snack foods, soups, canned meats, processed meats, cream substitutes and flavorings, ice cream, nuts, and so on. In other words, nearly all foods that are shelved, processed, refined, preserved, and not fresh can contain trans-fats.

The only way to eliminate them is to not consume any processed foods, and to make your own homemade condiments, soups, broths, etc., and by purchasing unprocessed 'real' foods.

Plants from which vegetable fats and oils are produced have evolved a variety of toxins designed by nature to protect them from 'predators' such as grazing animals, and their seeds contain a variety of toxins. The seed oils themselves block digestive enzymes that break down proteins in the stomach.

These digestive enzymes are necessary for proper digestion, production of thyroid hormones, clot removal, immunity and general adaptability of cells. Therefore using such plants to produce oils and fats is unnatural, and they are very damaging to the body.

From a nutritional standpoint, trans-fats provide no apparent benefit and can only be potentially harmful. The American Heart Association recommends that trans-fat consumption should be less than 1% of total daily calories (about 2 grams a day if based on a 2000 calorie per day diet), but optimally trans fats should be completely avoided.

Here are a few tips to knock toxic trans-fat out of your life:

- Read nutrition labels and stick to products that say they have zero grams of trans-fat. Then check the ingredients. If you notice 'partially hydrogenated oil' listed, put the product back on the shelf. These products may have up to 0.5 grams (FDA allows a product to say zero grams if it contains 0.5 or less).

- If you must buy a product with hydrogenated oil, be extra careful to only eat one serving - eat multiple portions and you are consuming a lot more trans-fat.
- Use olive or coconut oil or even butter when cooking at home rather than margarine.
- When dining out, avoid fried foods.

It is trans-fatty acid, as opposed to saturated fatty acid, consumption that is strongly correlated with cancer, cardiovascular disease, and other diseases. This is a volatile combination designed to extract and process oils, but it results in an extremely toxic product that the body only reacts to like it would to other toxins and poisons.

Several research centers in the United States have been developing a diet that can reverse hardening of the arteries (atherosclerosis). Some authorities now believe that this same diet may dramatically aid in prevention and treatment of heart disease, appendicitis, diverticular disease, gallstones, hypertension, varicose veins, deep vein thrombosis, pulmonary embolism, hiatus hernia, hemorrhoids, certain types of cancer, colitis and obesity.

This diet is a very natural diet. It is a vegetarian diet. It is low in fat and protein and high in complex carbohydrates such as potatoes, beans, corn, fresh fruit and most other unprocessed foods. Refined foods should be eliminated.

A natural food is one that comes with all its bulk and all its fiber plus all the vitamins and minerals. The vitamins and minerals exist so as to help metabolize and digest the natural food. Nature intended that we take in the bulk and the fiber plus the vitamins and the minerals and other nutrients all together to have a harmonious nutritional balance. When polyunsaturated fats are expressed from their natural parent foods, they need to be refined, deodorized, and even hydrogenated, depending on the food product for which they are used. In other words, most of the natural bulk is lost.

Foods that are not natural and not included in the diet include those that have been processed or have passed through a chemical factory. Examples abound. A walk through any supermarket will reveal aisle upon aisle of highly refined, over-processed foods which, unfortunately, are the mainstay of the American public's diet. The most prevalent, of course, are white sugar and refined (white) flour.

According to Archives of Internal Medicine, 1998, polyunsaturated fats increase a woman's risk of breast cancer by 69 %. In contrast, monounsaturated fats, as found in olive oil, reduce breast cancer risk by 45 %.

The total amount of fats in our diet today, according to the MAFF National Food Survey, is almost the same as it was at the beginning of this century; what has actually changed, to some extent, is the types of fats eaten. At the turn of the century we ate mainly animal fats that are largely saturated and monounsaturated. Now we are tending to eat more polyunsaturated fats – it is what we are advised to do. In 1991, two studies, from USA and Canada, found that linoleic acid, the major polyunsaturated fatty acid found in vegetable oils, increased the risk of breast tumors. This, it seems, was responsible for the rise in the cancers noted in previous studies.

Experiments with a variety of fats showed that saturated fats did not cause tumors but, when polyunsaturated vegetable oil or linoleic acid itself was added, it greatly increased the promotion of breast cancer. Cancer promotion is not the same as cancer causation. Promoters are the substances that help to speed up reproduction of already existing cancer cells.

In several studies, omega-6 linoleic acid appeared to be the crucial fatty acid. Vegetable oils (for example, corn oil and sunflower oil) which are rich in linoleic acid are potent promoters of tumor growth.

Body cell walls are made of cholesterol, protein and fats. The human body's fat make-up is largely of saturated and monounsaturated fatty acids. We contain very little polyunsaturated fat. Cell walls have to allow the various nutrients that body cells need from the blood and at the same time exercise a barrier function to harmful pathogens. They must be stable. An intake of large quantities of polyunsaturated fatty acids changes the constituency of cholesterol and body fat. Cell walls become softer and more unstable, in other words more liable to disease and cancer.

One study in mice has shown that consuming high amounts of polyunsaturated fat (but not monounsaturated fat) may increase the risk of metastasis in cancer patients. The researchers found that linoleic acid in polyunsaturated fats produced increasing membrane phase separation, and thereby increased adherence of circulating tumor cells to blood vessel walls and remote organs. According to the report, "the new findings support earlier evidence from other research that consuming high amounts of polyunsaturated fat may increase the risk of cancer spreading".

A study of 61,471 women aged 40 to 76, was conducted in Sweden to analyze the relation between different fats and breast cancer. The results were published in January 1998. This study found an inverse association with monounsaturated fat and a positive association with polyunsaturated fat. In other words, monounsaturated fats protected against breast cancer and polyunsaturated fats increased the risk. Saturated fats were neutral.

In today's nutritional world, fat has become a dirty word. Women in particular are encouraged to eat a low-fat diet to help prevent breast cancer, as well as other ailments, including other cancers. Animal fats such as butter have taken a terrible beating in the media over the past few decades and have been blamed for horrific crimes, including obesity, heart disease and cancer. Accordingly, Western people have been virtually brainwashed into thinking that butter and other predominantly saturated fats like coconut oil and tallow are unhealthy. So-called safe substitutes like margarine and various vegetable oils have been heavily promoted and advertised with the result being that the public associates these things with health and well-being.

141

Unfortunately for us, all of these contentions and claims are false. When it comes to breast cancer prevention, and in some cases treatment, the so-called 'bad fats' are actually the good guys, and the 'safe substitutes' are increasingly being shown up for what they really are: fabricated foods that cause disease, including breast cancer.

Flora margarine, the brand leader, is 39% linoleic acid; Vitalite and other 'own brand' polyunsaturated margarines are similar. Of cooking oils, sunflower oil is 50% and safflower oil 72% linoleic acid. Butter, on the other hand, has only a mere 2% and lard is just 9% linoleic acid.

Because of the heart disease risk from trans-fats in margarines, in 1994 the manufacturers of Flora changed its formula to cut out the trans-fats and other manufacturers have since followed. But that still leaves the linoleic acid.

In 3 out of 5 studies, the consumption of olive oil was associated with a significant decrease in the risk of breast cancer. Of the two remaining studies, one reported that the consumption of olive oil was associated with a lower incidence of breast cancer and the other reported no association between olive oil consumption and breast cancer. These studies were done in Mediterranean countries such as Greece, Italy and Spain, where women may have a total fat intake of about 42% of total calories. This total fat intake is comparable to or even higher than that seen in the U.S. However, the incidence of breast cancer is lower in these countries compared to the U.S. Although the total fat intake of these Mediterranean women is similar to that of American women, an important difference may be that most of the fat in their diets comes from olive oil. Humans have safely consumed olives and olive oil for thousands of years.

Researchers from the Catalonian Institute of Oncology (ICO) in Girona and the University of Granada in Spain have discovered that extra virgin olive oil appears to be a powerful weapon against breast cancer.

In a study just published in the scientific journal *BMC Cancer*, the scientists report that polyphenols - powerful natural antioxidants found in abundance in extra virgin olive oil (the least processed form of the oil) - have bioactivity against breast cancer cell lines.

In a review of olive oil research set for publication in the March edition of the journal *Critical Reviews in Food Science and Nutrition* (2009 Mar;49(3):218-36), scientists from Deakin University in Victoria, Australia, point out the health benefits of the so-called Mediterranean diet (such as a lower incidence of cardiovascular disease and atherosclerosis as well as several types of cancers) have been partially attributed to the regular consumption of virgin olive oil by Mediterranean populations.

The Australian researchers conclude this is likely due to the healthy physiological effects of virgin olive oil. For example, laboratory studies as well as those in humans and animals have shown that olive oil phenolics have a host of positive physiological effects, including preventing oxidative damage, quelling inflammation, regulating platelet and cellular function, and fighting infections.

Another interesting research, that throws light on the dangers of unhealthy polyunsaturated fats, has shown that out of 100 people who consumed large quantities of polyunsaturated fats, 78 showed marked clinical signs of premature aging. They also looked much older than others of the same age did. By contrast, in a recent study on the relationship between dietary fats and the risk for Alzheimer's disease, researchers were surprised to learn that the natural, healthy fats can actually reduce the risk for Alzheimer's by up to 80 %. The study showed that the group with the lowest rate of Alzheimer's ate approximately 38 grams of these healthy fats every day, while those with the highest incidence of this disease consumed only about half of that amount.

Although polyunsaturated fats appear to be more deceptively harmful, that does not mean it is okay to pound in saturated fats indiscriminately. A high saturated fat diet is also undesirable. Instead of having plenty of the low saturated fat containing sunflower oil, have olive oil or unsalted butter, and instead of that overly generous dollop, go a little easy. This way you're consuming the right fats in the right amounts. If your habits are good, you avoid tobacco and other addictives and of course if you control your PUFAs intake, you can relax knowing that your body is not hopelessly at the mercy of the ever-ready to ravage oxygen radicals. The tissue cells that have been damaged by abnormal free radical activity are unable to reproduce properly. This can impair major functions in the body, including those of the immune, digestive, nervous, and endocrine systems. Ever since refined polyunsaturated fats have been introduced to the population on a large scale during and after WWII, degenerative diseases have increased dramatically, skin cancer being one of them

Polyunsaturated fats have made sunlight 'dangerous', something that would never have been the case if foods hadn't been altered and manipulated, as they are today.

We now know that a bad diet full of polyunsaturated fats provides for an explosion of free radicals that we know are also unhealthy and disease-promoting. It is imperative, that we reduce the free radical onslaught by controlling our diet, cutting out the unnecessary polyunsaturates and consuming antioxidant-rich natural foods. There has to be a proper balance between the fats and antioxidants in our diet. This way we do not have to keep our toxic, sunlight-shy bodies hidden indoors and can freely step out into the shining glory that is the sun.

The colorful flower blooms brightly in the garden getting plenty of sunshine. The same flower in the darkness indoors withers and goes pale without the sun. Similarly the sun gives our skin color and richness. If we are deprived of it we turn pallid and dull. Even on the inside of our bodies. We only have to picture the little child playing in the sun all day, returning to a homemade, wholesome meal. This child is the epitome of youth and vigor, and owes his/her healthiness to sunlight and the right diet.

144

CHAPTER 14:
What Really Burns and Damages the Skin

A person who consumes polyunsaturated fats in his diet and exposes his skin to ultraviolet light to the point of reddening produces certain hormone-like substances called *prostaglandins* from the linoleic acid contained in the fats. Prostaglandins suppress the immune system, thereby contributing to tumor growth.

What is a prostaglandin?

A prostaglandin is any member of a group of lipid compounds that are derived enzymatically from fatty acids and have important functions in the animal body. Every prostaglandin contains 20 carbon atoms, including a 5-carbon ring. They are 'mediators' and have a variety of strong physiological effects, such as regulating the contraction and relaxation of smooth muscle tissue.

A study to investigate the relationship between sunlight UV radiation and diets containing varying amounts of polyunsaturated fats was performed. The study was conducted as follows.

A series of semi-purified diets containing 20% fat by weight, of increasing proportions (0, 5%, 10%, 15% or 20%) of polyunsaturated sunflower oil mixed with hydrogenated saturated cottonseed oil, was fed to groups of hairless mice during induction and promotion of photo-carcinogenesis. The photo-carcinogenic response was of increasing severity as the polyunsaturated content of the mixed dietary fat was increased, whether measured as tumor incidence, tumor multiplicity, progression of benign tumors to squamous cell carcinoma, or reduced survival. At the termination of the study approximately 6 months following the completion of the 10-week chronic UV irradiation treatment, when most mice bore tumors, the contact hypersensitivity (CHS) reactions in those groups supporting the highest tumor loads (fed 15% or 20% polyunsaturated fat), were significantly suppressed in comparison with the mice bearing smaller tumor loads (fed 0, 5% or 10% polyunsaturated fat). When mice were exposed acutely to UV radiation (UVR), a diet of 20% saturated fat provided almost complete protection from the suppression of CHS, whereas feeding 20% polyunsaturated fat resulted in 57% suppression; the CHS of unirradiated mice was unaffected by the nature of the dietary fat. These results suggest that the enhancement of photo-carcinogenesis by the dietary polyunsaturated fat component is mediated by an induced predisposition to persistent immunosuppression from chronic UV irradiation, and supports the evidence for an immunological role in dietary fat modulation of photo-carcinogenesis in mice.

The interesting point from this research is that the mice which were not given any polyunsaturated fats did NOT get skin cancers. In fact they appeared to be totally protected from skin cancer.

It was also found that as soon as they fed back polyunsaturated fats in a normal diet, the skin cancers appeared on all of the mice.

This result indicated that production of cancer cells are initiated but that somehow the absence of polyunsaturated fat interferes with the capacity of those potential cancer cells to grow out into full tumors. So an absence of polyunsaturated fat effectively inhibits the whole process of cancer development after sun exposure.

Some experiments have been carried out with a view to try and examine what happens in the later stage that controls whether the potential cancer cells shall develop or otherwise. The study yields that the genesis of cancer is possibly dependent upon prostaglandins which are formed from polyunsaturated fats in the body and if there is a deficiency in these prostaglandins the tumors fail to grow.

Polyunsaturated fat, whether it is eaten in low or high concentrations, seems to be associated with a higher risk of getting skin cancer. Remember the mice that didn't have any polyunsaturated fat and only a complete saturated fat diet were the ones that were protected. An equivalent approach in terms of human diet is a bit difficult because it is near impossible for a person to avoid all polyunsaturated fats. Nevertheless, if our intake of polyunsaturated fats is reduced considerably, it might also contribute to a reduction in the overall risk of skin cancer. Lower levels of polyunsaturated fat caused lesser or fewer lesions of skin cancers in mice than did high levels.

Health workers are now looking at alternative types of fats, for example fish oils. Fish oils contain an unusual type of super polyunsaturated fat which could replace the regular polyunsaturated fats in our diets. The prostaglandin equivalents which are produced from the fish oil type of polyunsaturates are different and have different bioactivity. Evidence from other research suggests that these different types are protective rather than stimulators of carcinogenesis. Researchers are looking at the possibility that the incorporation of fish oil into diet might have a protective function against skin cancer.

There is a whole range of prostaglandins and for every prostaglandin with one particular type of biological activity there is a counterpart that has the anti-activity. The human body has a very sophisticated mechanism for balancing one prostaglandin's activity against another. Prostaglandins together seem to be a vast regulatory mechanism which control many functions.

The role of prostaglandins in the development of cancer is not fully understood by scientists. It is suspected that they might be involved in immune regulation and somehow be caught up in the inability of the immune system to recognize and distinguish tumor cells. Tumor cells are foreign cells and under normal conditions the immune system would recognize and kill those cells. But when a tumor begins to grow successfully and unhindered, it implies that something has happened internally that has impaired the capacity of the immune system to identify and acknowledge the tumor cells as foreign entities that need to be attacked and done away with. It is likely that prostaglandins have a role to play in the process.

Yet another study suggests that prostaglandins are the most likely suspect involved in carcinogenesis. If those same mice are fed a drug called indomethacin, which inhibits the formation of prostaglandins from the polyunsaturated fats, the result is a remarkable protection from skin cancer.

There have been several studies performed to elicit how unsaturated fats inhibit enzymes and cause immune suppression.

According to researcher Peat, excessive unsaturated fats inhibit all body systems, mainly by inhibiting enzymes essential to metabolic processes required for health and immune protection and regulation. Here are some examples:

- Unsaturated fats directly kill white blood cells.
- Unsaturated oils inhibit proteolytic enzymes and this has far-reaching effects.
- Inhibition of proteolytic enzymes by unsaturated fats causes trouble at many sites where proteolytic enzymes are necessary such as-
- The digestion of dietary protein
- The digestion of clots
- The digestion of the colloidal protein released by the thyroid gland which leads to the active thyroid hormone production
- The digestion of cellular proteins involved in maintaining a steady state as new proteins are formed in the cell.

There is an enzyme system called the protein kinase C (PKC) system that is excessively activated by certain substances and certain conditions. Substances that cause excess activation of this system are: polyunsaturated fats (PUFAs), including free linoleic and linolenic acids, excess estrogen (a known cancer promoter) and cancer promoting phorbol esters.

These substances stimulate the cell while blocking the energy it needs to respond. The PKC system is also abnormally activated in diabetes and cancer. Unsaturated fats lead to thyroid suppression and consequent hormonal imbalances. Unsaturated oils block thyroid hormone secretion, its circulation and its tissue response. This leads to increased estrogen levels. The thyroid hormone is essential for the synthesis of the anti-aging hormones, namely pregnenolone, progesterone and DHEA. So when your thyroid is in trouble, the manufacture of these anti-aging steroids is correspondingly in trouble. Also, since thyroid converts cholesterol in your body to these anti-aging steroids, low thyroid function can lead to high cholesterol due to deficient cholesterol uptake or utilization for synthesis of certain steroid hormones.

Intravenous feeding with unsaturated fats is so powerfully immunosuppressive that it is now advocated as a way to prevent graft rejection (Mascioli, E., 1987). The poisonous effect of unsaturated fatty acids on the immune system has led to the development of new intravenous feeding products containing short and medium-chain saturated fats (Hashim, S., 1987).

Stress and hypoxia (oxygen deprivation) can cause cells to absorb large amounts of unsaturated fatty acids. It is now well accepted that cancer cells are dependent on unsaturated fatty acids for life and growth.

In 1927, Bernstein and Elias observed that a low unsaturated fat diet prevented the development of spontaneous tumors. Subsequent researchers have observed that unsaturated fats are essential for the growth of tumors. Tumors secrete a factor, which mobilizes unsaturated fats from storage, thus guaranteeing their supply in abundance until the fat tissues are depleted. In some experiments, the carcinogenic action of unsaturated fats was offset by adding thyroid glandular secretions. This observation suggests that at least part of the effect of unsaturated oils is to inhibit thyroid function.

149

Ip et al. (1985) studied the relationship of carcinogenicity to the percentage of unsaturated fats ranging from 0.5% to 10%. His results show that the optimum unsaturated fat intake may be 0.5% or less. In addition to inhibiting the thyroid gland, unsaturated fats impair intercellular communication, suppress several immune functions related to cancer, and are present at high concentrations in cancer cells, where their antiproteolytic action would be expected to interfere with the proteolytic enzymes and to shift the equilibrium towards growth. Even though cancer cells are known to have a high level of unsaturated fats, they have a low level of lipid peroxidation. Since lipid peroxidation inhibits growth, there is an absence of growth restraint in these cancer cells. Not only this, but as has been mentioned above, tumor cells also exhibit a function that ensures their perpetuation, that is, they are capable of secreting a substance which mobilizes (releases) unsaturated fats insuring a continual, steady supply from the fat stores in the body until all of it has been exhausted.

Consumption of unsaturated fats has been associated with both skin aging and with the sensitivity of the skin to ultraviolet damage. According to Black (1985), ultraviolet light-induced skin cancer is mediated by unsaturated fats and lipid peroxidation.

If your body is already subjected to an overdose of free radicals courtesy dietary unsaturated oils and you add sunscreens to your skin, you have the perfect combination - a dangerous chemical cocktail - to produce skin cancer, especially on areas more exposed to the sun than others.

As has been explained in the previous chapter, edible oils never occur in large quantities in nature. To obtain one tablespoon of corn oil in natural form you would have to eat 12-18 ears of corn. Since oil extraction from corn, grains, and seeds became possible 80-90 years ago, consumption of polyunsaturated and unsaturated fats (thicker oils) as salad and cooking oils has increased dramatically in the industrialized world.

150

The very basic difference between a healthy person's way of looking at vegetable oils and the industrial oil technician's viewpoint should be clearly understood. When the technician sees dark color, it represents the presence of 'impurities' - material that prevents the oil from being light colored, odorless and bland in taste. From a healthy knowledgeable person's viewpoint, those 'impurities' are entirely desirable. Why? Simply because the very things which impart color, odor and flavor are nothing but nutrients. It is a real tragedy and even paradoxical that the removal of nutrients should be equated with 'purity'. It is a tragedy because, if those very nutrients were present, they would contribute to the health of the consumer and not the other way around. And it is a bit of paradox because establishing the desired 'purity' as they call it, actually results in producing poor quality food.

There are three methods of extracting vegetable oils from nuts, grains, beans, seeds or olives. The first is by use of a hydraulic press. This is an ancient method and yields the best quality oil, retaining the highest concentration of the original nutrients. The only two materials that will yield enough oil without heating them first before pressing are sesame seeds and olives. Therefore, sesame oil and olive oil from a hydraulic press are the only oils which could truly be referred to as 'cold pressed' oils. Unfortunately the term 'cold pressed' and 'virgin' are meaningless to the common consumer. They have no legal definition and mean whatever the manufacturer wants them to mean. They do not give a true description of the product behind the label. The term 'virgin' for olive oil rightfully refers only to the first pressing by a hydraulic press without heat. The term 'cold pressed' refers only to hydraulic pressing without heat. These oils are the closest possible to the natural state, therefore have the most color, odor and flavor. They are the most nutritive and the least degraded. Sadly these kinds of oils are often unavailable because too little is produced in this way.

If an oil has been extracted by hydraulic press but has been heated prior to pressing, it is to be referred to as 'pressed' and not 'cold pressed'.

The second method is by expeller. This method uses a screw or continuous press with a constantly rotating worm shaft. Cooked material goes into one end and is put under continuous pressure until it is discharged at the other end with oil squeezed out. Temperatures between 200 and 250 degrees are normal. Obviously, this type of extraction does not qualify as 'cold pressed' either, it is referred to as expeller pressed.

Now, with a hydraulically pressed oil, labeled 'cold pressed' or 'pressed', you can assume that you have crude or unrefined oil. But this is not true of 'expeller pressed' oil because the common fate of expeller pressed oil is to be refined after extraction. However expeller pressed crude or unrefined oils may be obtained and are healthier that those which undergo refining.

The last method is solvent extraction, which is outright hazardous to health. Oil bearing raw materials are ground, steam cooked, then mixed with the solvent (of a petroleum base) which dissolves out of the oils, leaving a dry residue. The solvent is separated from the oils later on. This method is universally used by the big commercial oil processors because it gets more oils out quicker and cheaper. About 98% of the soy oil in the U.S. is solvent extracted.

The most commonly used solvents are light petroleum fractions. The four types of Naptha used are Pentane, Heptane, Hexane, and Octane. Another solvent used is synthetic Trichlorethylene. Some of these chemicals are commonly found in gasoline. The most used solvent is Hexane. Oils dissolved and extracted by this method are solvent extracted dissolved oils and not pressed oils.

The big commercial edible oil processors and distributors tell us that if any of the solvent remains in the oils it is only very little. But you must know just how harmful these solvents may be. Pertinent here is an

152

observation coming from a symposium of cancer specialists organized by the International Union Against Cancer meeting in Rome in August 1956. Among many things they observed: "Since various petroleum constituents, including certain mineral oils and paraffin, have produced cancer in man and experimental animals, the presence of such chemicals in food appears to be objectionable, particularly when such materials are heated to high temperatures.

The 'very little' argument for solvent residues is just as weak for solvents used for oil extraction as it is for pesticide residues. The amount of petroleum solvents that should enter the human system is zero!

Refining is usually accomplished with the addition of sodium hydroxide and temperatures around 450 degrees. The oil after this initial process in refining is not considered edible without further processing, such as filtration, deodorization, bleaching etc. According to the Encyclopedia Britannica refined oils are "low in color (thinner) and more susceptible to rancidity". Where bleaching is concerned, they say: "Physical absorption methods involve treating hot oils with activated carbons, fuller's earths or activated clays. Many impurities including chlorophyll and Vitamin A are absorbed onto the agents and removed by filtration. Bleaching by any of these means reduces the resistance of oils to rancidity."

Here is an industry which regards precious nutrients as 'impurities'. Not just the chlorophyll and Vitamin A, but also the Vitamin E and phosphorous compounds such as lecithin, too. Then they further compound an already thoroughly compounded felony by virtually guaranteeing that the oil will turn rancid unless of course they load the product with preservative - which of course is always done. The only exception would be in the case of the so-called 'health food' oils which are poor quality and low-nutrition but are at least preservative-free and have to be refrigerated to avoid rancidity.

It has been found that the digestion of oils is clearly retarded by rancidity. The products of rancidity were found to be lethal to rats. The degenerative diseases caused by rancid oils are undoubtedly brought about by the destruction of vitamins E, F, and A, both in the oil itself and in the body.

Oil processing is so effective at making the end result free of odor and flavor that it is even possible for rancid oil to be 'reclaimed' and sold for human consumption. There is no proof that this is actually done but it is all the same an open possibility. Unfortunately this is the era of industrialized foods. Good nutrition is almost given no consideration at all. What is more important to the manufacturer is the privilege of controlling large quantities of foods at large profits. They must protect the pocket, not the person.

Health and natural food store operators have in almost all cases not been able to advise the consumer because they have been misled too. It has been discovered that oils which have been solvent extracted, refined, bleached and deodorized have been sold as 'cold pressed'. Knowing these facts, no one genuinely interested in good nutrition should now continue to be a party to the hoax.

The process of refining oils is exactly analogous to the refining of whole wheat and whole sugar into white 'pure' varieties. In all cases, a raw product full of natural vitamins, minerals, enzymes and other food factors is taken and then the original natural food is cruelly reduced into a relative 'nonfood' – devitalized and stripped of all nutrition.

One thing that may not be clear and probably will be asked is- What keeps crude oils from going rancid, especially in stores that handle them in bulk as well as the bottled ones? The answer is that crude oils, being unrefined, retain their natural anti-oxidants which prevent rancidity. How can one test it just to be sure? One drop on the tongue is sufficient to tell the story - rancidity is so bitingly, bitterly sharp and it is absolutely unmistakable. However that should be looked upon as a good thing because this way you have a simple household quality test that relies on your own sensory faculty and does not need to be lab-analyzed to ascertain quality. If you have been cheated into using refined oils, it would be impossible for you to tell if the oil in your kitchen is spoiled and rancid, it will remain the same- tasteless, odorless and colorless.

Of course, when one has been accustomed to bland, virtually tasteless refined oil, the introduction of crude oil into the diet means experiencing the 'real thing'. This experience of reality is due to the fact that for the first time you shall taste oil which contains all its natural vitamin A, all its natural vitamin E, all its natural lecithin, and all of the other natural food factors. When you come to appreciate the facts, as a consumer, it will be easy to accept a superior food irrespective of the taste it may impart in cooking.

It is interesting to know that the average person today consumes polyunsaturated fats 16 times more than a person did 90 years ago. That does not include all the other types of fats contained in today's foods.

The diets of most North Americans and Europeans have dramatically changed over the last 30 years. Refined vegetable oil, specifically soybean oil, is now being used in most snack foods, breads, sweets, and processed foods to such an extent approximately 20% of the total caloric intake is estimated to come from this source alone.

Why is this so dangerous for our health?

Refined vegetable oil, like soybean oil or Canola oil, is an omega-6 fatty acid. Our body needs fats to survive, but many nutritional experts believe that to achieve optimal health, humans need to balance their fat intake between omega-6 fatty acids, derived from seeds and nuts, and omega-3 fatty acids, primarily found in Chia Seeds, flax seeds, walnuts and almonds (and also in cold water fish such as salmon, sardines, herring, and mackerel). Vegetable preparations like baked winter squash, broccoli, cauliflower, spinach, Brussels sprouts and cabbage, also contain good amounts of omega-3 fats. Today instead of a 1:1 balanced

155

intake of omega-6 and omega-3 fatty acids, most western diets contain anything between a 10:1 and a 50:1 ratio of omega-6 to omega-3 fatty acids. Radically changing that ratio is the best thing we can do at the present moment to change the future of our health.

Increased omega-6 intake can be attributed to obesity, depression, hyperactivity, and possibly even violence. Omega-6 fatty acids increase inflammation at the cellular level, which may explain the rise in hypertension, heart disease, certain types of cancers, asthma, and cognitive degenerative diseases. Omega-3 fatty acids on the other hand are precursors for anti-inflammation agents and help counterbalance the negative effects from the high levels of omega-6 fats we consume every day in our diets.

Simple changes to our diets to reduce our omega-6 fatty acid intake may be difficult due to the wide ranging use of soybean oils in processed foods. The best bet to reduce your omega-6 fatty acid intake is to avoid processed foods in favor of freshly prepared meals that contain those above mentioned foods.

Lack of exercise, fresh air, and foods rich in nutrients make it even less possible for a human being to cope with large amounts of unnatural fats.

Unlike most animals, humans are a relatively high fat diet-eating species. Rats and mice eat foods containing about 5% fat, mostly from grains that contain about 2 or 3% fat. Rabbits, deer, moose, caribou, sheep, goats, African cattle, horses, and zebra consume foods containing less than 1% fat. Carnivorous wild dogs, wolves, and wild cats have about 5% fat in their diets, because their prey is lean, averaging about 3% body fat.

Very few animals eat high fat diets. Carnivorous birds occasionally eat high fat fish. Whales that eat salmon get about 10 to 15 % fat from that diet. Bears enjoy a similar diet for a short time in fall, but consume low fat foods the rest of the year.

Traditionally, humans consumed 15-20 % of their calories as fats and oils. This is far less than the 40 % fat from present-day refined oils, grease-laden convenience foods, trans-fatty-acid-containing margarines, shortenings, and partially hydrogenated vegetable oils, fat spreads, and fat-inbred pork and beef.

Not only must the right amount (15-20 %) of fats and oils be present in a diet appropriate for human health, but they must also be the right kind and quality of fats and oils. We must choose between those that heal and those that kill.

Although polyunsaturated refined oils are unhealthy, it does not mean that naturally occurring PUFAs are also dangerous. In fact in adequate amounts, they are essential fatty acids (EFAs). The polyunsaturated fats that heal effectively are fresh, unprocessed fats containing one or both EFAs. EFAs are rather like vitamins - they were once referred to as vitamin F.

We must remember that if fat soluble vitamins are in excess, the body fails to excrete them and this leads to a state of hypervitaminosis (vitamin excess) which is unhealthy and undesirable. Similarly, essential fatty acids need to be taken in only requisite amounts. If they are in excess, the consequences are disagreeable. Nevertheless in appropriate amounts, EFAs are every bit as important to health as protein, vitamins, and minerals.

Both types of EFAs - linoleic acid (LA) and linolenic acid (LNA) have vital functions in all cells. Both are extremely sensitive to destruction and become toxic with exposure to light, oxygen, frying, or hydrogenation. To promote good health, both EFAs must be present, in their natural state and in adequate quantities, in our diet. I stress here again that it is not possible and one should not attempt to deprive the body completely of polyunsaturates. Their deficiency can also give rise to health problems.

Lack of Linoleic Acid can cause the following deficiency symptoms that resemble so many degenerative disease of the 20th century:

157

- Eczema-like skin eruptions
- Hair loss
- Liver degeneration
- Behavioral disturbances
- Kidney degeneration
- Excessive water loss through the skin
- Excessive thirst
- Susceptibility to infections
- Failure to heal wounds
- Male sterility
- Miscarriage
- Arthritis-like conditions
- Heart and circulatory problems
- Retarded growth

LA deficiency is of course relatively rare, because our intake of LA has escalated drastically during the last 50 years, due to increased intake of polyunsaturated oils, mainly corn and safflower.

If anything, our intake of LA is too high. Although it is essential to health, we must not forget that excessive consumption of LA can promote tumor growth and cancer.

Lack of LNA can cause several deficiency symptoms such as:

- Retarded growth
- Weakness
- Impaired vision and learning
- Loss of motor coordination
- Tingling sensation in arms and legs
- Behavioral changes
- Lack of LNA can also result in:
- High serum triglycerides
- High blood pressure
- Sticky platelets
- Tissue inflammation

158

- Water retention (edema)
- Dry skin
- Mental deterioration
- Low metabolic rate
- Some kinds of immune dysfunction

The best sources of EFAs are seeds and nuts that contain them in their natural, unspoiled form, along with protein, minerals, vitamins, and fiber and fresh, unrefined oils or blends carefully pressed in the absence of light and air, shelf-dated, and kept in dark brown (or opaque) glass bottles.

For every step we take in processing away from the natural state of whole, fresh, raw, sun-ripe, organic, in-season and locally grown, something of value is lost from food. For this loss, we pay a price in health. This is also true for oils.

The majority of commercial manufacturers begin with cheap and/or rotten, discarded, broken, inedible seeds, and from these they make the refined, bland, tasteless, odorless, colorless oils in clear glass and plastic bottles that adorn the marketplace.

Let us review the events in refining here. The oil is treated with sodium hydroxide - as in corrosive sink and drain cleaners, then with phosphoric acid - as in corrosive window washing acid that cuts grease. Then it is bleached and deodorized at a destructively high temperature.

During these processes, most of the beneficial minor ingredients are removed, and small amounts (perhaps 1% of the oil weight) of many toxic substances are formed. The oil changes from protective against mutations (unrefined) to mutation-causing (refined). Oil to margarine! Having removed the minor ingredients and having produced toxic substances, we subject the refined oils to a further insult called hydrogenation, carried out at frying temperature for 6 to 8 hours to make margarines (cheap imitation butter) and shortenings (to replace lard) as well as partially hydrogenated vegetable oils (to give body to potato chips, other junk foods, candy, and bakery products). In this process, the essential nutrients of LA and LNA are selectively and systematically destroyed. Trans-fatty acids are formed in large quantities, and they make up from 9 to 50 % of the total in most hydrogenated products. In addition, other unnatural toxic products are formed. This processing is a remarkable destruction of a whole, nutrient-rich, natural food with many health benefits.

The only conclusion that can be drawn is that the effect of oil consumption on human health has taken a 180 degree turn and the common man silently suffers unaware of the crimes committed by industries.

We can categorize the fats that kill into four groups:

- Hydrogenated and partially hydrogenated oils
- Fried oils
- Refined commercial vegetable oils
- Hard fats (relatively benign)

Hydrogenated and partially hydrogenated oils include margarine, shortenings, shortening oils and partially hydrogenated vegetable oils that are used in junk foods, convenience foods, candies, confections, cookies, breads, and other baked products.

The EFAs in these products have been largely destroyed and converted into toxic products that increase cholesterol levels and promote cancer and atherosclerosis. The largest group of these toxic substances, trans-fatty acids, makes up twice the amount of all other food additives combined. The trans-fatty acids have detrimental effects on:

- Cardiovascular function (they increase bad LDL, decrease good HDL, make platelets stickier, and double the risk of heart attack)
- Some aspects of the immune system
- Insulin response and function (detrimental for diabetics)

160

- Liver function (inhibit detoxification)
- Reproductive function
- Pregnancy
- Birth weight (low)
- Breast milk quality
- Cell membranes
- EFA functions

Fried oils have been subjected to the destructive effects of light, air (oxygen), and high temperature, all at the same time. EFAs are destroyed in hundreds of different possible ways, resulting in a mixture of toxic molecules. Fried oils have been shown to increase both atherosclerosis and cancer.

Frying is a health-destroying practice, no matter what fat or oil is used. The more EFAs an oil contains, the more toxic it becomes when fried. For those unwilling to give up this health-destroying practice, small amounts of butter cause the least damage to health, but also provide no EFAs, which must come from fresh, unrefined oils in brown glass bottles.

Refined oils are those which have been overheated, producing some toxic molecules. And of course, beneficial minor ingredients including vitamin E, carotene, lecithin, and phytosterols, have been removed.

Our bodies can deal with some hard fats, but an excess of hard or saturated fats makes platelets stickier, slows metabolic rate, results in fat deposition and weight gain, interferes with insulin function and interferes with the function of EFAs.

So what is the conclusion? Small amounts of saturated fats are part of our natural diet. Refined oils, fried oils and partially hydrogenated oils found in margarines, shortenings, and convenience foods are unnatural food additives to be avoided. Unnatural fats impair the digestive power and lead to a build-up of toxins and subsequent crises of toxicity. The presence of excessive amounts of free radicals indicates that the body is full of toxins.

161

Once they infiltrate the skin tissue, even short-term exposure to ultraviolet light can burn and damage skin cells. If your eyes and skin are sensitive to sunlight, this indicates that your body is toxic.

Your body has the natural capacity to inform you when something within your system is deranged. It is a simple feedback mechanism. When something is amiss, your body throws out signs and symptoms which tell you that attention is needed. With careful observation and deduction and without rash medical interference you will realize that most of your problems arise from simple deficiencies and excesses. And these problems can only completely be overcome by adding where there is too little and subtracting where there is too much. The body functions optimally when it is optimally balanced.

If your eyes and skin are sensitive to sunlight you need to clean out the internal toxicity. Flush out the over-accumulated toxins. Subsequent efforts to avoid the sun may result in serious light deficiency, which can lead to serious health problems. You would end up only compounding one excess with another deficiency and further upsetting your health. To avoid sunlight in such a situation would be an attempt at quelling the effect of the original affection instead of treating the essential cause. It would be a wasted if not dangerous exercise.

The UV light entering through the eyes is known to stimulate the immune system. Today, more than 50% of the U.S. population wears prescription or sun-protective glasses, which are able to block out most UV light. The latest fashion is to wear plastic glasses, which also block out all UV light. The same holds true for plastic contact lenses. Indoor activities, sunscreens, clothing, UV-repelling windows, etc. make certain that we receive very little of it.

Without regular exposure to sunlight, however, the immune system decreases its effectiveness with every year of age.

162

With sunlight, the use of oxygen in the body tissues increases, but without it, our cells begin to starve for oxygen. This leads to cellular malfunction, premature aging, and even death. Starved of a balanced sunlight diet, we tend to look for help elsewhere, even though nature is ready to cure us at any time.

It is very unfortunate that sick people are mostly kept indoors, often with curtains drawn and windows closed. One of nature's most potent preventive and curative powers is there for everyone to use.

CHAPTER 15:
Guidelines for Increasing Sun Exposure

It has by now become clear in your mind that sunlight is as vital a necessity for life and health as is air, food and water. You have also come to realize how beneficial sunlight can prove to be in both the prevention and cure of ever so many common diseases and dreadful illnesses too.

It is a nutrient, a medicine, a remedy all at once. It is not some bottled compound you can find at a drug store alone. It is naturally available to everyone. The dosage is under your control and your body easily tells you when you have had just about the right amount of it.

Even though sunlight is readily available all through the day, some people fail to profit from it because of limiting life situations. Typically a sedentary lifestyle, a 9 to 5 job that keeps you rooted to the desk for the most part of the day through the most part of the week, for instance. The quantum of solar energy your cells can soak up is profoundly diminished this way. However the situation can certainly be helped as there are definite ways to increase your exposure to the sun in a less direct manner than the more obvious outdoor activities.

If you wish to benefit from the sun and cannot afford much time to be outdoors, some of the many ways by which you can increase your exposure to sunlight even while indoors include the following:

- Windows should be made of glass that permits UV light to enter
- Have as many such windows as possible
- Keep your curtains pushed back so that you have maximum exposure
- Depending on the weather and the season, keep your windows open
- Install as many full spectrum lights as possible (the best alternative to natural sunlight)

People living in a moderate climate can sunbathe regularly. It is best to avoid the sun between 10.00 a.m. and 3.00 p.m. during summers when the UV concentration in sunlight is too high and hot infra-red rays predominate, contributing to a feeling of discomfort and uneasiness. If for any reason you anticipate sun exposure for unduly long periods, you may apply Aloe Vera gel, coconut oil, or olive oil. For maximum benefits, though, and to wash off any natural oiliness, it is best to take a shower before sunbathing. Aloe Vera is known to be particularly effective in sunburn cases. It is often referred to as 'the burn plant' and works wonders on all types of burns, especially sunburns. Aloe Vera contains lignins which are chemical compounds that form an integral part of the cell walls. Lignins help the skin to heal faster.

Aloe Vera also works as an effective pain reliever, acting as a cooling agent on the surface. It also contains salicylic acid, the same pain-killing agent found in aspirin. Aloe Vera also contains two chief compounds - gibberellins and glycans which have effective anti-inflammatory properties.

Virgin coconut oil and olive oil are particularly effective in the treatment of sunburns being natural moisturizers and exfoliants.

During winter, spring, and fall, it is alright to expose yourself to the noonday sunlight that you would otherwise have chosen to avoid in the summer, as it is far milder. In fact it is often so that during winter mornings and evenings the sunlight intensity is insufficient, and noonday exposure is quite beneficial.

People often think that sunbathing is an activity that should be restricted to the summer months only. This is not true. It is very much possible to sunbathe even during cold winters, provided you lie in a totally wind protected place. The idea is to get some sun without the chill.

165

You can build your own sunbathing area against a wall facing the sun. The sidewalls should be made of material that can serve as a good windbreak. The wall pointing toward the sun should be at an angle slanted toward the sun so that the low slanting winter rays can shine into the sunbathing area and sufficiently illuminate it.

Lying on a blanket, you will find that you feel warmer than you did indoors.

Another, perhaps, more practical way is to open a window on a sunny day without breeze. I have done this many times in my life, even in countries where winters can be very cold.

When sunbathing is practiced for health reasons and not for a mere cosmetic purpose, it is very important to have a phased beginning - at first restricting yourself to shorter periods avoiding chances of burns and then gradually increasing the length of exposure and eventually tuning your exposure consciously to a sufficient extent regularly.

The civilized human has long forgotten how to respond to sudden extreme changes in surrounding physical elements. This is because we have discovered ways to cheat nature's seasonal variations and regulate our living environment with genius technologies indeed. The resultant lack of flexibility has lead to poor adaptability to environmental variations. It is therefore often dangerous to suddenly thrust the body into a completely new environment. Instead, a phased exposure over a period of time proves to be a more wise and practical approach. The same must be kept in mind when starting up a sunbathing regimen.

Start your sunlight treatment by exposing your entire body (if possible) for a few minutes, and then increase the time each day by a few more minutes until you reach 20-30 minutes. Alternatively, walking in the sun for 40-60 minutes several times a week has similar benefits. This will give you enough sunlight to keep your body and mind healthy, provided you incorporate the basic measures of a balanced diet, lifestyle, and daily routine as outlined in *Timeless*

166

Secrets of Health and Rejuvenation. Your body can store a certain amount of vitamin D, which may last you through 4-6 weeks of wintry weather, but it is always good to recharge your 'vitamin D battery' whenever possible by exposing yourself to direct sunlight.

Note: Avoid conventional sunlamps, tanning beds, and tanning booths. According to a study published in the *International Journal of Cancer* (Vol 120, No 5, March 1, 2007; 1116-1122), exposure to tanning beds before age 35 increases melanoma risk by 75 %. Many young people now use tanning beds, which may be responsible for the recent sharp increase of melanomas in their age group. There is also a link between tanning bed use and squamous cell carcinoma, a less deadly type of skin cancer. Conventional tanning equipment uses *magnetic ballasts* that emit powerful electromagnetic fields (EMFs) responsible for cancer growth. Their high concentration of UVA may also play a role. Electronic ballasts are much safer than magnetic ballasts, but very few parlors use these.

I personally recommend the SunSplash Renew System (large standing UV light) offered at Dr. Mercola's web site, www.mercola.com. I use one myself during the cold winter months. Smaller, vitamin D lamps (UV lamps) offered on the Internet, are also safe and effective in keeping Vitamin D levels balanced during the cold season.

Please note: As a rule of thumb, if the shadow of your body (while you stand in the sun) appears to be longer than your body height, the UVB radiation from the sun is too weak to induce vitamin D production in your skin.

Also, after sunbathing avoid using soap to wash your skin, except in the private areas and under the arms. Water is fine. Soap removes all the layers of oil containing the vitamin D your body has produced during sun exposure. It takes up to 48 hours for the body to absorb all the vitamin D it has produced. Of course, avoid sunscreens, otherwise the body will not make any Vitamin D at all.

CHAPTER 16:
The Ancient Practice of Sun Gazing

The ancient people of almost every culture and religion knew that sunlight was the key to immortality and enlightenment. The ancient Incas, Egyptians, Hindus, Zoroastrians, Essenes, Greeks, Romans, Chinese, and Native Americans would gaze at the sun during certain times of the day, recite special prayers and mantras, and perform various rites. Most traditional archaeologists and anthropologists dismiss this as the customary sun worship of primitive societies. They ignore the fact that the monotheistic solar religions of Zarathustra and Akhenaton liberated people for a short while from bondage to the superstitions of pantheistic religions and created peaceful Utopian societies. They also forget that the great old teacher of sun gazing, Lord Meru, otherwise known as El Dorado or Quetzalcoatl, raised the primitive tribes of the Central and South American jungles into civilized societies that had knowledge of medicine, metallurgy, farming, animal husbandry, writing, engineering, mathematics and astronomy with cities containing hundreds of stone buildings, water and sewer systems and paved roads. Scientists and historians fail to realize that the physical sun was only the outer symbol of the object of worship, which was in truth, the spiritual Sun behind the physical sun which can enlighten people and transform them into beings of light.

Sun energy is the source that powers the brain. It enters the body through the elements of air, water, fire, and earth. Sunlight enters and leaves the human body most easily and directly through the human eye, provided it isn't filtered out by colored lenses. The eyes are the grand portals through which sunlight enters the body.

Sun gazing is an ancient practice that can induce healing of body and mind.

The eyes are very complex organs, consisting of 5 billion parts intricately designed and functioning in unity. The primary function of the eye is light-dark perception.

Even the most basic, simplest 'eyes', such as those belonging to unicellular organisms have no other function but to detect whether the surroundings are light or dark in order to maintain the circadian rhythms.

Acting as a photo lens, the human eye is able to break down the entire spectrum of sunlight into the different color rays - a sort of ocular prism. In a camera, the various rays of light react with the chemicals of the film and encode the pictures you take accordingly. Likewise, upon entering the pineal gland in the brain, the different light rays are chemically encoded in the brain and passed on to the organs and systems in the body.

The vital organs of the body are dependent on specific colors of the light spectrum. For kidney cells to function properly, for example, they require red light. Heart cells need yellow light, and liver cells require green light. Light deficiencies in any of the organs and systems of the body can lead to disease. Regular sun gazing can help restore balance and efficiency to all cells in the body.

The pineal gland is one of the most researched glands of the body. Scientists have established that bright light stimulates the production of serotonin and melatonin in the pineal, but there are other neurochemicals produced by the pineal that have more profound and complex effects apart from regulation of moods, sleep, reproductive function and body temperature.

Scientists at the University of Pennsylvania, including Dr. George C. Brenarr, a leading authority on the pineal gland, observed the sun yogi HRM (Hira Ratan Manek) for 130 days in 2002. They found that his pineal exhibited growth and reactivation. The average size of the pineal is 6×6 mm, but in HRM's case it was 8×11 mm.

Scientists refer to the pineal gland as the 'atrophied third eye'. Indeed, it, along with the pituitary, is the third eye chakra or energy center, better referred to as dormant rather than atrophied. According to Max Heindel's Rosicrucian writings, in the distant past, man was in touch with the inner

169

worlds through an activated pineal and pituitary gland. Considered the most powerful and highest source of ethereal energy available to humans, the third eye has always been important in initiating psychic powers (clairvoyance and seeing auras etc).

To activate the 'third eye' and perceive higher dimensions, the pineal and the pituitary must vibrate in unison, which is achieved through meditation or sun gazing. When a correct relationship is established between the personality operating through the pituitary, and the soul operating through the pineal, a magnetic field is created. The pineal can generate its own magnetic field because it contains magnetite. This field can interact with the earth's magnetic field. The solar wind at dawn, charging the earth's magnetic field, stimulates the pineal gland. This is why many spiritual teachings claim that the period between 4 and 6 am is the best time to meditate and why sunrise is the best time to sun gaze. At these times, the pineal stimulates the pituitary to secrete Human Growth Hormone. That is why sun gazers often experience rapid nail and hair growth, restoration of hair color, and general rejuvenation. Cleopatra used to place a magnet on her forehead to stimulate the pituitary to restore her youth and good looks. She did not know she already had a magnet in her head.

The technique of sun gazing demands no more than time and attention, and is very simple. One should gaze at the sun only in the morning or evening hours, about one hour or less after sunrise or before sunset. Look at the rising or setting sun once a day. On the first day, look at the sun in a relaxed manner for a maximum of 10 seconds. On the second day, look at it for 20 seconds, adding about ten seconds every succeeding day. After ten continuous days of sun gazing you will be looking at the sun for about 100 seconds. The eyes can blink or flicker and don't need to be steady. To receive the main benefits of sun gazing, you need to increase the duration in the above manner until you reach three months.

This brings you up to the length of 15 minutes of gazing at a time.

At this stage, the sun energy of the sun's rays passing through the human eye will be charging the hypothalamus tract - the pathway behind the retina leading to the human brain. As the brain increasingly receives extra power through this pathway, you will find a drastic reduction of mental tension and worries. With access to this additional source of energy, you are likely to develop a more positive mindset and increased self-confidence. If you suffer from anxieties and depression, you will find that these go away. Sadness and depression are known to increase with reduced or lack of exposure to sunlight. With fewer worries and fears, your brain may use the saved and additionally supplied energy for healing and improvement of mental and physical wellbeing.

One of the most frequently reported benefits of regular sun gazing is improvement of eyesight.

Life giving, golden rayed, the eternal watchful eye, called 'the beginning' and 'the ultimate truth' by wisdom, the Sun, is also the earliest acknowledged doctor of mankind. We have turned to him for healing since ages - since our very beginnings.

About Andreas Moritz

Andreas Moritz is a medical intuitive; a practitioner of Ayurveda, iridology, shiatsu, and vibrational medicine, a writer, and an artist. Born in southwest Germany in 1954, Andreas had to deal with several severe illnesses from an early age, which compelled him to study diet, nutrition and various methods of natural healing while still a child.

By age 20, he had completed his training in both iridology - the diagnostic science of eye interpretation - and dietetics. In 1981, Andreas began studying Ayurvedic medicine in India and finished his training as a qualified practitioner of Ayurveda in New Zealand in 1991. Rather than being satisfied with merely treating the symptoms of illness, Andreas has dedicated his life's work to understanding and treating the root causes of illness. Because of this holistic approach, he has had great success with cases of terminal disease where conventional methods of healing proved futile.

Since 1988, he has practiced the Japanese healing art of shiatsu, which has given him insights into the energy system of the body. In addition, he has devoted eight years of research into consciousness and its important role in the field of mind/body medicine.

Andreas Moritz is also the author of *Timeless Secrets of Health & Rejuvenation, The Amazing Liver and Gallbladder Flush, Cancer Is Not a Disease! — It's A Survival Mechanism, Lifting the Veil of Duality, It's Time to Come Alive, Heart Disease No More!, Simple Steps to Total Health, Diabetes - No More!, Ending the AIDS Myth, Heal Yourself with Sunlight* and *Hear The Whispers, Live Your Dream.*

During his extensive travels throughout the world, Andreas has consulted with heads of state and members of government in Europe, Asia and Africa, and has lectured widely on the subjects of health, mind/body medicine, and spirituality. His popular *Timeless Secrets of Health &*

Rejuvenation workshops have assisted people in taking responsibility for their own health and well-being. Andreas has had a free forum '*Ask Andreas Moritz*' on the large health website, curezone.com (five million readers and increasing). Although he has stopped writing for the forum, it contains an extensive archive of his answers to thousands of questions on a variety of health-related topics.

Since taking up residence in the United States in 1998, Andreas has been involved in developing a new and innovative system of healing called Ener-Chi Art that targets the root causes of many chronic illnesses. Ener-Chi Art consists of a series of light ray-encoded oil paintings that can instantly restore vital energy flow (Chi) in the organs and systems of the body. Andreas is also the founder of Sacred Santémony - Divine Chanting for Every Occasion, a powerful system of specially generated frequencies of sound that can transform deep-seated fears, allergies, traumas, and mental or emotional blocks into useful opportunities for growth and inspiration within a matter of moments.

Other Books by the Author

The Amazing Liver and Gallbladder Flush
A Powerful Do-It-Yourself Tool
to Optimize Your Health and Wellbeing

In this internationally bestselling Andreas Moritz addresses the most common but rarely recognized cause of illness—gallstones congesting the liver. Although those who suffer an excruciatingly painful gallbladder attack are clearly aware of the stones congesting this vital organ, few people realize that hundreds if not thousands of gallstones (mainly clumps of hardened bile) have accumulated in their liver, often causing no pain or symptoms for decades.

Most adults living in the industrialized world, and especially those suffering a chronic illness such as heart disease, arthritis, MS, cancer, or diabetes, have gallstones blocking the bile ducts of their liver. Furthermore, 20 million Americans suffer from gallbladder attacks every year. In many cases, treatment consists merely of removing the gallbladder, at the cost of $5 billion a year. This purely symptom-oriented approach, however, does not eliminate the cause of the illness, and in many cases, sets the stage for even more serious conditions.

This book provides a thorough understanding of what causes gallstones in both the liver and gallbladder and explains why these stones can be held responsible for the most common diseases so prevalent in the world today. It provides the reader with the knowledge needed to recognize the stones and gives the necessary, do-it-yourself instructions to remove them painlessly in the comfort of one's own home. The book also shares practical guidelines on how to prevent new gallstones from forming. The widespread success of *The Amazing Liver and Gallbladder Flush* stands as a testimony to the strength and effectiveness of the cleanse itself. This powerful yet simple cleanse has led to extraordinary improvements in health and wellness among thousands of people who have already given themselves the precious gift of a strong, clean, revitalized liver.

Timeless Secrets of
Health and Rejuvenation
Breakthrough Medicine for the 21st Century
(550 pages, 8 ½ x 11 inches)

This book meets the increasing demand for a clear and comprehensive guide that can helps people to become self-sufficient regarding their health and wellbeing. It answers some of the most pressing questions of our time: How does illness arise? Who heals, and who doesn't? Are we destined to be sick? What causes aging? Is it reversible? What are the major causes of disease, and how can we eliminate them? What simple and effective practices can I incorporate into my daily routine that will dramatically improve my health?

Topics include: The placebo effect and the mind/body mystery; the laws of illness and health; the four most common risk factors for disease; digestive disorders and their effects on the rest of the body; the wonders of our biological rhythms and how to restore them if disrupted; how to create a life of balance; why to choose a vegetarian diet; cleansing the liver, gallbladder, kidneys, and colon; removing allergies; giving up smoking, naturally; using sunlight as medicine; the "new" causes of heart disease, cancer, diabetes, and AIDS; and a scrutinizing look at antibiotics, blood transfusions, ultrasound scans, and immunization programs.

Timeless Secrets of Health and Rejuvenation sheds light on all major issues of healthcare and reveals that most medical treatments, including surgery, blood transfusions, and pharmaceutical drugs, are avoidable when certain key functions in the body are restored through the natural methods described in the book. The reader also learns about the potential dangers of medical diagnosis and treatment, as well as the reasons vitamin supplements, "health foods,"

175

low-fat products, "wholesome" breakfast cereals, diet foods, and diet programs may have contributed to the current health crisis rather than helped to resolve it. The book includes a complete program of healthcare, which is primarily based on the ancient medical system of Ayurveda and the vast amount of experience Andreas Moritz has gained in the field of health restoration during the past 30 years.

Cancer is Not a Disease –
It's A Survival Mechanism
Discover Cancer's Hidden Purpose, Heal its Root Causes, and be Healthier Than Ever!

In *Cancer is Not a Disease,* Andreas Moritz proves the point that cancer is the physical symptom that reflects our body's final attempt to deal with life-threatening cell congestion and toxins. He claims that removing the underlying conditions that force the body to produce cancerous cells, sets the preconditions for complete healing of our body, mind, and emotions.

This book confronts you with a radically new understanding of cancer – one that revolutionized the current cancer model. On the average, today's conventional "treatments" of killing, cutting out, or burning cancerous cells offer most patients a remission rate of a mere 7%, and the majority of these survivors are "cured" for just five years or fewer. Prominent cancer researcher and professor at the University of California at Berkeley, Dr. Hardin Jones, stated: "Patients are as well, or better off, untreated..." Any published success figures in cancer survival statistics are offset by equal or better scores among those receiving no treatment at all. More people are killed by cancer treatments than are saved by them.

Cancer is Not a Disease shows you why traditional cancer treatments are often fatal, what actually causes cancer, and how you can remove the obstacles that prevent the body from healing itself. Cancer is not an attempt on

176

your life; on the contrary, this "dread disease" is the body's final, desperate effort to save your life. Unless we change our perception of what cancer really is, it will continue to threaten the life of nearly one out of every two people. This book opens a door for those who wish to turn feelings of victimhood into empowerment and self-mastery, and disease into health.

Topics of the book include:

- Reasons the body is forced to develop cancer cells
- How to identify and remove the causes of cancer
- Why most cancers disappear by themselves, without medical intervention
- Why radiation, chemotherapy, and surgery never cure cancer
- Why some people survive cancer despite undergoing dangerously radical treatments
- The roles of fear, frustration, low self-worth, and repressed anger in the origination of cancer
- How to turn self-destructive emotions into energies that promote health and vitality
- Spiritual lessons behind cancer

Lifting the Veil of Duality
Your Guide to Living without Judgment

"Do you know that there is a place inside you – hidden beneath the appearance of thoughts, feelings, and emotions – that does not know the difference between good and evil, right and wrong, light and dark? From that place you embrace the opposite values of life as *One*. In this sacred place you are at peace with yourself and at peace with your world." - *Andreas Moritz*

In *Lifting the Veil of Duality*, Andreas Moritz poignantly exposes the illusion of duality. He outlines a simple way to remove every limitation that you have imposed upon yourself during the course of living in the realm of duality. You will be prompted to see yourself and the world through a new lens – the lens of clarity, discernment, and non-judgment. You will also discover that mistakes, accidents, coincidences, negativity, deception, injustice, wars, crime, and terrorism all have a deeper purpose and meaning in the larger scheme of things. So naturally, much of what you will read may conflict with the beliefs you currently hold. Yet you are not asked to change your beliefs or opinions. Instead, you are asked to have *an open mind,* for only an open mind can enjoy freedom from judgment.

Our personal views and worldviews are currently challenged by a crisis of identity. Some are being shattered altogether. The collapse of our current world order forces humanity to deal with the most basic issues of existence. You can no longer avoid taking responsibility for the things that happen to you. When you *do* accept responsibility, you also empower and heal yourself.

Lifting the Veil of Duality shows you how you create or subdue your ability to fulfill your desires. Furthermore, you will find intriguing explanations about the mystery of time, the truth and illusion of reincarnation, the oftentimes misunderstood value of prayer, what makes relationships work, and why so often they don't. Find out why injustice is an illusion that has managed to haunt us throughout the ages. Learn about our original separation from the Source of life and what this means with regard to the current waves of instability and fear so many of us are experiencing.

Discover how to identify the angels living amongst us and why we all have light-bodies. You will have the opportunity to find the ultimate God within you and discover why a God seen as separate from yourself keeps you from being in your Divine Power and happiness. In addition, you can find out how to heal yourself at a moment's notice. Read all about the "New Medicine" and the destiny of the old medicine, the old economy, the old religion, and the old world.

It's Time to Come Alive!
Start Using the Amazing Healing Powers of Your Body, Mind, and Spirit Today!

In this book, the author brings to light man's deep inner need for spiritual wisdom in life and helps the reader develop a new sense of reality that is based on love, power, and compassion. He describes our relationship with the natural world in detail and discusses how we can harness its tremendous powers for our personal and humanity's benefit. *It's Time to Come Alive* challenges some of our most commonly held beliefs and offers a way out of the emotional restrictions and physical limitations we have created in our lives.

Topics include: What shapes our destiny; using the power of intention; secrets of defying the aging process; doubting – the cause of failure; opening the heart; material wealth and spiritual wealth; fatigue – the major cause of stress; methods of emotional transformation; techniques of primordial healing; how to increase the health of the five senses; developing spiritual wisdom; the major causes of today's earth changes; entry into the new world; 12 gateways to heaven on earth; and many more.

Simple Steps to Total Health!
Andreas Moritz with co-author John Hornecker

By nature, your physical body is designed to be healthy and vital throughout life. Unhealthy eating habits and lifestyle choices, however, lead to numerous health conditions that prevent you from enjoying life to the fullest. In *Simple Steps to Total Health*, the authors bring to light the most common cause of disease, which is the build-up of toxins and residues from improperly digested foods that inhibit various organs and systems from performing their normal functions. This guidebook for total health provides you with simple but highly effective approaches for internal cleansing, hydration, nutrition, and living habits.

The book's three parts cover the essentials of total health – Good Internal Hygiene, Healthy Nutrition, and Balanced Lifestyle. Learn about the most common disease-causing foods, dietary habits and influences responsible for the occurrence of chronic illnesses, including those affecting the blood vessels, heart, liver, intestinal organs, lungs, kidneys, joints, bones, nervous system, and sense organs.

To be able to live a healthy life, you must align your internal biological rhythms with the larger rhythms of nature. Find out more about this and many other important topics in *Simple Steps to Total Health.* This is a "must-have" book for anyone who is interested in using a natural, drug-free approach to restore total health.

Heart Disease No More!
Make Peace with Your Heart and Heal Yourself
(Excerpted from Timeless Secrets of Health and Rejuvenation)

Less than one hundred years ago, heart disease was an extremely rare illness. Today it kills more people in the developed world than all other causes of death combined. Despite the vast quantity of financial resources spent on finding a cure for heart disease, the current medical approaches remain mainly symptom-oriented and do not address the underlying causes.

Even worse, overwhelming evidence shows that the treatment of heart disease or its presumed precursors, such as high blood pressure, hardening of the arteries, and high cholesterol, not only prevents a real cure, but also can easily lead to chronic heart failure. The patient's heart may still beat, but not strongly enough for him to feel vital and alive.

Without removing the underlying causes of heart disease and its precursors, the average person has little, if any, protection against it. Heart attacks can strike whether you have undergone a coronary bypass or had stents placed inside your arteries. According to research, these procedures fail to prevent heart attacks and do nothing to reduce mortality rates.

Heart Disease No More, excerpted from the author's bestselling book, *Timeless Secrets of Health and Rejuvenation*, puts the responsibility for healing where it belongs, on the heart, mind, and body of each individual. It provides the reader with practical insights about the development and causes of heart disease. Even better, it explains simple steps you can take to prevent and reverse heart disease for good, regardless of a possible genetic predisposition.

Diabetes--No More!
Discover and Heal Its True Causes
(Excerpted from Timeless Secrets of Health and Rejuvenation)

According to this bestselling author, diabetes is not a disease; in the vast majority of cases, it is a complex mechanism of protection or survival that the body chooses to avoid the possibly fatal consequences of an unhealthful diet and lifestyle.

Despite the body's ceaseless self-preservation efforts (which we call diseases), millions of people suffer or die unnecessarily from these consequences. The imbalanced blood sugar level in diabetes is but a symptom of illness, not the illness itself. By developing diabetes, the body is neither doing something wrong, nor is it trying to commit suicide. The current diabetes epidemic is man-made, or rather, factory-made, and, therefore, can be halted and reversed through simple but effective changes in diet and lifestyle. *Diabetes—No More* provides you with essential information

181

on the various causes of diabetes and how anyone can avoid them.

To stop the diabetes epidemic you need to create the right circumstances that allow your body to heal. Just as there is a mechanism to become diabetic, there is also a mechanism to reverse it. Find out how!

This book was excerpted from the bestselling book, *Timeless Secrets of Health and Rejuvenation.*

Ending the AIDS Myth
It's Time to Heal the TRUE Causes!
(Excerpted from Timeless Secrets of
Health and Rejuvenation)

Contrary to common belief, no scientific evidence exists to this day to prove that AIDS is a contagious disease. The current AIDS theory falls short in predicting the kind of AIDS disease an infected person may be manifesting, and no accurate system is in place to determine how long it will take for the disease to develop. In addition, the current HIV/AIDS theory contains no reliable information that can help identify those who are at risk for developing AIDS.

On the other hand, published research actually proves that HIV only spreads heterosexually in extremely rare cases and cannot be responsible for an epidemic that involves millions of AIDS victims around the world. Furthermore, it is an established fact that the retrovirus HIV, which is composed of human gene fragments, is incapable of destroying human cells. However, cell destruction is the main characteristic of every AIDS disease.

Even the principal discoverer of HIV, Luc Montagnier, no longer believes that HIV is solely responsible for causing AIDS. In fact, he showed that HIV alone could not cause AIDS. Increasing evidence indicates that AIDS may be a toxicity syndrome or metabolic disorder that is caused by immunity risk factors, including heroin, sex-enhancement drugs, antibiotics, commonly prescribed

AIDS drugs, rectal intercourse, starvation, malnutrition, and dehydration.

Dozens of prominent scientists working at the forefront of AIDS research now openly question the virus hypothesis of AIDS. Find out why! *Ending the AIDS Myth* also shows you what really causes the shutdown of the immune system and what you can do to avoid this.

Hear the Whispers, Live Your Dream
A Fanfare of Inspiration

Listening to the whispers of your heart will set you free. The beauty and bliss of your knowingness and love center are what we are here to capture, take in and swim with. You are like a dolphin sailing in a sea of joy. Allow yourself to open to the wondrous fullness of your selfhood, without reservation and without judgment.

Judgment stands in the way, like a boulder trespassing on your journey to the higher reaches of your destiny. Slide these boulders aside and feel the joy of your inner truth sprout forth. Do not allow another's thoughts or directions for you to supersede your inner knowingness, for you relinquish being the full, radiant star that you are.

It is with an open heart, a receptive mind, and a reaching for the stars of wisdom that lie within you, that you reap the bountiful goodness of mother Earth and the universal I AM. For you are a benevolent being of light and there is no course that can truly stop you, except your own thoughts, or allowing another's beliefs to override your own.

May these aphorisms of love, joy and wisdom inspire you to be the wondrous being that you were born to be!

Feel Great, Lose Weight

No rigorous workouts. No surgery. In this book, celebrated author Andreas Moritz suggests a gentle – and permanent – route to losing weight. In this ground-breaking book, he says that once we stop blaming our genes and take control of our own life, weight-loss is a natural consequence.

"You need to make that critical mental shift. You need to experience the willingness to shed your physical and emotional baggage, not by counting calories but by embracing your mind, body and spirit. Once you start looking at yourself differently, 80 per cent of the work is done."

In Feel Great, Lose Weight, Andreas Moritz tells us why conventional weight-loss programs don't work and how weight-loss 'experts' make sure we keep going back. He also tells us why food manufacturers, pharmaceutical companies and health regulators conspire to keep America toxically overweight.

But we can refuse to buy into the Big Fat Lie. Choosing the mind-body approach triggers powerful biochemical changes that set us on a safe and irreversible path to losing weight, without resorting to crash diets, heavy workouts or dangerous surgical procedures.

All books are available paperback and as electronic books through the Ener-Chi Wellness Center

Website: http://www.ener-chi.com
Email: support@ener-chi.com

Toll free 1(866) 258-4006 (USA)
Local: 1(709) 570-7401 (Canada)

INDEX

A

Acetaminophen, liver injury by, 80
Acral lentiginous melanoma, 65
ACS. *See* American Cancer Society
Acute photo-toxicity, 123
Adaptation
    cold environments, 25
    definition, 24
    hot climates, 25–26
    humid climates, 25
Advertising campaigns
    cigarette smoking, 55
    sunscreen, 32
African Americans
    melanoma patients, survival
        rate of, 66
    skin cancer risk in, 65
        migration to colder climates
            and, 66–67
Age and drug hepatotoxicity, link
    between, 80
Air, 3
Air-conditioning, health problems
    associated with, 60–63
Alcohol consumption and
    hepatotoxic drugs, 81
Aloe Vera, 165
American Cancer Society, 100, 101
Animal fats
    myths associated with, 141
Antarctic ozone hole, 17
Antibodies, cloaking of, 28
Artificial light and cancer risk, link
    between, 63–64
Avobenzone, 47

B

Balanced diet
    importance of, 120, 122
    sunlight, 73
Basal cell carcinoma (BCC), 12
Benign tumors, 11

Benzophenone, 41
Beverages, dehydration due to, 70
Bimolecular reactions,
    chromophore and DNA, 40
Bi-specific complexes, 28
Bisphosphonate drugs, kidney
    damage risk, 82
Blood pressure
    geographic and racial
        differences in, 113
    regulation by vitamin D, 92
    ultraviolet-induced vitamin D
        synthesis impact on, 114
Body, human
    absorption of UV light, 76
    composition of, 70
    dependence on colors of light
        spectrum, 169
    feedback mechanism, 162
    self-regulating mechanisms, 26,
        77–78
Bone loss and vitamin D
    concentration, relation
    between, 94
Breast cancer risk
    polyunsaturated oils and, 140
    prevention with vitamin D, 99–
        100, 101
    sunscreen use and, 52
Breastfed baby, vitamin D
    supplementation in, 96, 97
Butter, 132, 133
    ingredients of, 131

C

Calamine lotion, 36–37
Calciferol. *See* Vitamin D
Calcium and vitamin D
    supplements, 100
Cancer. *See also* Breast cancer risk
    causes of, 11
        exposure to artificial light,
        63
        nuclear testing, 56

characterization of, 11
genesis of, 146
mortality
    and latitude, link between, 99
    and UVB light levels, link between, 84
treatment by
    moving to areas of higher UV-concentration, 34
    UVA light, 28
    UVB radiation, 27
types of, 11
Carcinogenesis. *See also* Cancer
genetic material abnormalities, 11
prostaglandins role in, 147, 148
unsaturated fat role in, 149, 150
Carcinogens, 11
Cardiovascular disease (CVD) risk factors, 116
Cell walls, body
barrier functions, 141
composition of, 140
Chemical sunscreens. *See* Sunscreens
Chlorine and ozone destruction, link between, 16
Chlorofluorocarbons (CFCs) and ozone depletion, 15–16
CHS. *See* Contact hypersensitivity
Clinical trials, 78
Cloaking, antibodies, 28
Coconut oil, 132, 133
Cod liver oil, 93
Cold environments, physiological variations in, 25
Cold pressed oil, 151
Colon cancer
risk with high-fat diets, 103
vitamin D protection against, 102, 103
Congestive heart failure, 91
Conjugated linoleic acid, 133
Contact hypersensitivity, 145, 146
Cosmetic industry, 57

Cosmic rays, 4
Cough reflex, 35
Crude oils, 154
Cutter Biological, 57
Cytochrome P450 enzyme system, 79

D

Desert-adapted person, adaptation of, 25–26
Diabetes mellitus type 1
blood sugar levels after sun exposure, 116
prevalence of, 115
risk and sunlight exposure, relation between, 115, 116
vitamin D and, 93, 105
Disease
causes of, 9
cure and, 9
DNA
absorption spectrum of, 38
internal conversion, 38, 39
photo-protective mechanism, 39
DNA damage
direct and indirect, 38
    sunscreens and, 40–41
free radicals and ROs role in, 37, 38
PABA role in, 43
Doshas, 68
pitta body, 68–69
Drug
clinical trials, 78
hepatotoxicity of
    dose-dependent, 79–80
    factors influencing, 80–82
    idiosyncratic reaction, 80
    liver injury, 78
-induced photosensitivity. *See* Photosensitivity reactions
withdrawn due to liver injury, 79
Dry environment and body moisture, 61

186

E

EFAs. *See* Essential fatty acids
Electromagnetic waves, 4
Essential fatty acids, 134, 135
    functions of, 157
    hydrogenated and partially
        hydrogenated oils, 160
Exercise/exercising in Sun, 107
    blood pressure reduction, 114
    guidelines for, 111
    heart efficiency and, 115
    hypertension treatment with,
        114
    reducing stress levels, 117
    significance of, 107, 108
    testosterone release
        stimulation, 111
Expeller pressed oil, 152
Eye diseases
    incidence in industrialized
        world, 77
    sunglass uses and, 76
Eyes, functions of, 168, 169

F

Fats
    breast cancer and, relation
        between, 141
    consumption of
        animal, 156
        human, 157
    misconception about, 128
    unsaturated. *See* Unsaturated
        fats
Fatty acids
    classification of, 128
    definition of, 128
    EFAs. *See* Essential fatty acids
    harmful effects
        omega-6 and omega-3 fatty
            acids, 156
        unsaturated fatty acids, 149
    source of, 133
    TFA. *See* Trans-fatty acid
Fibromyalgia, 106

Fish oils, 147
Flora margarine, 142
Fluorescent lighting, harmful
    effects of
    higher stress levels, 60
    melanoma risk, 32, 59
Food and Drug Administration
    drug approval, 78
    light therapy approval, 27
    PABA ester approval, 44
Food chain and sunlight, 2
Foods, 2
Free radicals, 37
    cell damage by, 127, 144
    DNA damage by, 39, 41
    generation by sunscreen
        chemicals, 54, 55
    generation from
        polyunsaturated fats, 126,
        127, 129, 144
Fried oils, harmful effects of, 161

G

Gazing to Sun. *See* Sun gazing
Genetic material abnormalities and
    cancer development, 11
Gymnasia, ill-effects of, 108

H

HCl and ozone destruction, link
    between, 16
Heart attack, risk with vegetable
    oils and margarines, 130
Heart efficiency, exercise and
    sunbathing influence on, 115
Heliotherapy, 6
    health benefits of, 7–8
Hepatitis C and hepatotoxic drugs,
    81
High altitudes and UV radiation,
    link between, 24
HIV and drug hepatotoxicity, 81
Hormone production and UV-rays,
    9

187

Hot climates, physiological
    variations in, 25
Human breast milk
    synthetic vitamin D2 in, 98
    vitamin D deficiency in, 96, 97
Human skin. *See* Skin, human
Humid climates, physiological
    variations in, 25
Hydrogenated oils, 160
Hypertension
    geographic and racial
        differences in, 113, 114
    prevalence of, 113
    prevalence of, 114
Hypogonadism, 110

I

Immune system
    effect of underexposure to
        sunlight on, 65
    stimulation by sunlight
        exposure, 162
Incandescent light, exposure to, 65
Indoor lifestyle
    damage to body cells by, 76
    skin cancer risk with, 32–33, 59,
        60
    tips to increase sunlight
        exposure, 164
Indoor exercise, 108
    ill-effects of, 109
Infertility problems and sunlight
    exposure, link between, 112
Inflammations
    skin cancer relation with, 13
    vitamin D and, 90, 92
Insulin action, short-term exercise
    impact on, 116
Interferons, MS treatment using,
    86
Internal conversion, 38, 39
Intravenous feeding with
    unsaturated fats, 149

K

Kidney damage
    associated with bisphosphonate
        drugs, 82
    drug hepatoxicity and, 81

L

LA. *See* Linoleic acid
Lassitude, 121
LCA. *See* Lithocholic acid
Light therapy
    cancer treatment by
        lung cancers, 29
        UVA light, 28
        UVB radiation, 27
    depression treatment, 117
    infertility treatment, 113
    menstrual cycle normalization,
        112
Linoleic acid
    deficiency symptoms, 158
Linoleic acid
    high intake and cancer risk,
        136, 140
    sources of, 159
Lithocholic acid, 102
Liver injury drug-induced, 78–80
Lung cancer risk
    smoking and, 29
    underexposure to sunlight and,
        28, 29

M

Malignant melanoma. *See also* Skin
    cancer
    causes of, 13
        DNA damage, 41
        sunscreen use, 50–51
        UVA radiation, 20
    clinical features of, 12, 13
    diagnostic definition, 33
    early detection of, 13
    incidence of, 13, 21, 33

188

office workers and
outdoors, 59
Queensland, 36
risk factors
indoor fluorescent lights, 32
sunscreen ingredients, 40,
49
sites for, 34
Margarines
heart attack risk with, 130
ingredients of, 132
manufacturing process, 131
Medical professionals and
misconceptions about sunlight
diagnostic definition of
melanomas, 33
sunlight/melanoma link, 31
Mediterranean diet, health
benefits of, 143
Melanin, 39
lifetime of, 40
pitta body types and, 71
Menopause and osteoporosis, 94
Menstrual problems and sunlight
exposure, link between, 112
Metastasis, 11
Methotrexate, hepatotoxicity of,
81
5-Methoxypsoralen (5-MOP),
harmful effects, 45–46
Monounsaturated fats, 126
breast cancer and, relation
between, 141
source of, 128
MS. *See* Multiple sclerosis
Multiple sclerosis
clinical features of, 85–86
autoimmune condition, 89
vitamin D deficiency, 103,
104
mortality and sun exposure,
relation between, 89–90
prevalence of, 29
treatments
interferons, 86
vitamin D, 87–88, 105

UV exposure and, relationship
between, 29–30
Musculoskeletal function and
vitamin D, relationship
between, 118, 119

N

Natural food, 139
Night cold, 25
Nighttime illumination and cancer
risk, link between, 63–64
Non-melanomas, 13

O

Obesity
drug hepatotoxicity and, link
between, 82
vitamin D utilization
impairment, 106
Olive oil, 132
breast cancer prevention with,
142
extraction using hydraulic
press, 151
Omega-6 and omega-3 fatty acid
intake, harmful effects of, 156
Ornithine decarboxylase (ODC)
activity, 45
Osteoporosis, 94, 105
Outdoor jobs and skin cancer risk,
link between, 59
Overexposure to sun, 9
indications of, 35
suppressing, 22, 51
Oxidative stress, 37, 127
Oxybenzone, 42
Oxygen, importance of, 126
Oxygen free radicals, 126, 127
Ozone, 6
concentration measurements,
limitations to, 17
depletion
CFCs role in, 15–16
malignant melanoma and,
20

189

skin cancer relation with,
15–16
UVB radiation and, 17–18

P

PABA. *See* Para-amino-benzoic acid
Padimate O, 44
Para-amino-benzoic acid, 43
Partially hydrogenated oils, 160
Pathogenic bacteria
    drug-resistant strains and
        drugs, 9
    killing using UV, 1
Petroleum constituents in edible
    oil, 152
Phenytoin, 80
Photo-carcinogenesis by
    polyunsaturated fat, 145, 146
Photophobia, 76
Photo-protection, 39
Photosensitivity reactions
    photoallergic reactions, 123
        skin manifestations of, 124
    phototoxic reactions
        causes of, 122
        nail manifestations of, 124
        skin manifestations of, 123,
        124
Photosensitizing drugs, 124
Pigmentary changes, 124
Pineal gland
    atrophied third eye, 169, 170
    stimulation by light, 169
Pitta body type, 68
    characteristics of, 68, 69
    exposure to sun, 71–72
    sunscreens adverse effect in, 71
Polyunsaturated fats, 144
    breast cancer risk with, 140,
    141
    cooking, 129
    metastasis risk with, 141
    premature aging with, 143
    rancidity of, 126, 129
    refined oils and, 134
    skin cancer risk with, 146, 147

sources of, 128
Prostaglandins
    definition of, 145
    role in carcinogenesis, 147, 148
Prostate cancer
    artificial lighting and, link
        between, 63–64
    vitamin D deficiency and, 101,
    102
Protein kinase C (PKC) system,
    substances causing excess
    activation of, 148, 149
Protests, nuclear weapons testing,
    56
Pseudoporphyria, 124
Psoralen-containing sunscreens
    ban on, 44
Psoralen (ultraviolet light-activated
    free radical generator), 44
PUFAs. *See* Polyunsaturated fats
Punta Arenas, 17

R

Reactive oxygen species
    definition of, 37
    harmful effects of, 38
Refined vegetable oil
    harmful effects of, 156, 161
    omega-6 fatty acid content, 155
Refining process
    filtration, deodorization,
        bleaching, 153
    harmful effects of, 155, 159,
    160
    hydrogenation, 159
Rickets, 105
    causes for rise of infant, 96
    characterization of, 95
ROS. *See* Reactive oxygen species

S

SAD. *See* Seasonal affective
    disorder
Saturated fats, 126
    cooking, 132

190

functions of, 135
ill-effects of diet containing
    high, 143
nutrients and substances in,
    132
sources of, 128
stability of, 128
SCC. *See* Squamous cell carcinoma
Seasonal affective disorder, 107
Sesame oil, 126
Skin aging, 150
Skin cancer
    causes of, 11
        UV sources, 13, 15, 20, 51
    diet and, relation between, 120,
        121
    incidence of, 14, 18, 19, 32
    skin inflammation relation with,
        13
    sunscreens and, link between,
        49
    types of, 12–13
Skin cancer rates
    global restrictions on ozone
        depleting agents and, 19–20
    Northern European countries,
        10
Skin, human
    absorption of sunscreen
        ingredients, 42
    damage, 21
    factors influencing effect of sun
        on, 14
    lack of moisture in, 60–61
    photo-protection of, 39
Skin pigmentation, desert-adapted
    people, 26
Smoking and lung cancer risk, 29
Solar energy, 1, 168
    stored in plants, 2
    uses of, 3
Solar radiation
    types of, 6
    ultraviolet light. *See* Ultraviolet
        light
Solitrol, functions of, 10
SPF. *See* Sun protection factor

Squamous cell carcinoma, 12
Sun
    electromagnetic waves, 4
    influence on earth's climate and
        seasonal changes, 3
    overexposure to. *See*
        Overexposure to sun
    supporting growth of species, 3
    worship in civilizations and
        cultures, 3–4
Sun gazing, 168
    benefits of, 171
    technique of, 170
Sunbathing
    avoiding soap use after, 167
    phased beginning of, 166
    risk with fats and processed
        foods, 120
    suntan lotions and malignant
        skin cancer risk, 42
Sunburn, 49
    signs and skin damage, 21
Sunglasses, 8
    use and eye diseases, 76, 77
Sunlight exposure
    cancer treatment by, 34
    health benefits of, 73, 106, 107,
        108, 117
    immune stimulating effects, 1
    misconception about, 5, 35
        medical professionals
            challenging, 31, 33
        skin diseases, 21
    summer season, 165
    winter, spring, and fall season,
        165
Sunning, eyes, 77
Sun protection factor, 46
Sunscreens, 31
    blocking UV rays, 36
    Calamine lotion, 36–37
    concerns associated with uses
        of, 49–50
    EWG study of, 47, 48
    ingredients
        absorption into skin, 42
        avobenzone, 47

191

benzophenone, 41
cancer risk, 54
free radicals and ROS
    generation by, 37, 42, 54
melanoma risk, 50–51
5-MOP, 45–46
PABA, 43
psoralen, 44
UV filter, 39
primary defects of, 55
protection against UVB
    radiation, 46, 48, 50
skin cancer risk and, 32, 36, 49,
    52
SPF claims, 48
tin oxide, 36
vitamin D deficiency due to,
    52–53
Sun System III (SS III), 45, 46
Suntan lotions
ban on, 45
malignant skin cancer risk of, 42
Sun tanning, 117
Synthetic vitamin D, 106

T

Tanning beds, melanoma risk with
    exposure to, 167
Testosterone
bio-available (free) levels of,
    110
guidelines for maximizing
    effects of exercise on, 111
sunlight exposure impact on,
    109, 110
TFA. See Trans-fatty acid
Thermal adaptations, 25
Thirst disease, 70
Thyroid hormone secretion
metabolism and, 9
unsaturated fats and, 149
Tin oxide as reflecting coating, 36
Trans-fatty acid
characterization of, 136
harmful effects of, 137, 160
sources of, 137, 138

tips for eliminating, 138, 139
Tuberculosis treatment using UV
    light, 7, 8
Type 1 Diabetes. See Diabetes
    mellitus type 1

U

Ultraviolet germicidal irradiation,
    74–75
Ultraviolet light, 5
characterization of, 6
DNA damage by, 38
effect of hypothetical increase
    in, 23
germicidal frequency of, 15
health benefits of, 74
hemoglobin and, 10
influence on life forms, 4
intensity variation, 6
    higher altitudes, 24
    poles and equator, 23
    wavelength, 75
manmade sources of, 6
measurements in United States,
    18–19
multiple sclerosis, relationship
    between, 29–30
skin cancer, link between, 20,
    51
solitrol activation, 10
sterilization using, 1, 74
thyroid gland stimulation by, 9
UVA radiation
    melanoma induction by, 20
    side-effects of blocking, 71
UVB radiation
    cancer treatment using, 27
    lung cancer risk, link
        between, 29
    ozone variations and, 17–18
    researcher's claim on rise in,
        18
    side-effects of blocking, 71
Underexposure to sunlight,
    harmful effects of
    infertility, 112

192

lung cancer risk, 28
menstrual periods, 112
mental and physical problems,
    9–10
risk factor for cancer, 84
skin cancer, 10
starvation for oxygen, 163
Unhealthy oils, 121
Unsaturated fats. *See also*
    Polyunsaturated fats
    carcinogenic action of, 149, 150
    enzyme inhibition by, 148
    hormonal imbalances due to,
        149
    immunosuppression by, 149
    lipid peroxidation of, 150
UVGI. *See* Ultraviolet germicidal
    irradiation
UV lamps, 119, 167

biologic function of, 85
breast cancer risk and, 99–100
calcium concentration
    regulation, 91–92
diabetes mellitus and, 93
dietary sources of, 85, 95–96
different forms of, 85
multiple sclerosis prevention
    by, 87–88
musculoskeletal disease and, 94
role in healthy heart, 92
steroid hormone precursor, 97
Vitamin D receptor
    binding with LCA, 103
    gene polymorphisms, 101

V

Vegetable oils
    extraction methods
        expeller and solvent
            extraction, 152
        hydraulic press, 151
        petroleum constituents in, 152,
            153
        rancidity of, 154
        refining of, 153, 154
        view of healthy person and
            technician on, 151
Vegetarian diet, 139
Virgin olive oil, health benefits of,
    142
Vitamin D deficiency
    causes of, 92
    diseases and conditions caused
        by, 105
    heart disease and
        congestive heart failure, 91
        inflammation, 90–91
    risk in young adults during
        winter, 97–98
    sunscreen use and, 51, 52–53
Vitamin D, 117

W

Water drinking, importance of, 70,
    120

193

Lightning Source UK Ltd.
Milton Keynes UK
UKOW04f2320020115

243906UK00001B/42/P